www.wadsworth.com

wadsworth.com is the World Wide Web site for Wadsworth and is your direct source to dozens of online resources.

At *wadsworth.com* you can find out about supplements, demonstration software, and student resources. You can also send email to many of our authors and preview new publications and exciting new technologies.

wadsworth.com
Changing the way the world learns®

CHISELED
IN
SAND

Perspectives on Change in
Human Services Organizations

~

Robert Cohen
Virginia Commonwealth University

Jessye Cohen

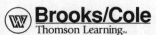
Brooks/Cole
Thomson Learning™

Australia • Canada • Denmark • Japan • Mexico • New Zealand • Philippines
Puerto Rico • Singapore • South Africa • Spain • United Kingdom • United States

Counseling Editor: *Lisa Gebo*
Assistant Editor: *Susan Wilson*
Editorial Assistant: *JoAnne vonZastrow*
Marketing Assistant: *Jessica McFadden*
Project Editor: *John Walker*
Print Buyer: *Mary Noel*
Permissions Editor: *Susan Walters*

Production Service: *Janet Vail*
Copy Editor: *Heath Silberfeld*
Text and Cover Designer: *John Walker*
Cover Images: *PNI*
Cover Printer: *Webcom*
Compositor: *Janet Vail*
Printer/Binder: *Webcom*

For more information, contact
Wadsworth/Thomson Learning
10 Davis Drive
Belmont, CA 94002-3098
USA
www.wadsworth.com

International Headquarters
Thomson Learning
290 Harbor Drive, 2nd Floor
Stamford, CT 06902-7477
USA

UK/Europe/Middle East
Thomson Learning
Berkshire House
168-173 High Holborn
London WC1V 7AA
United Kingdom

Asia
Thomson Learning
60 Albert Street #15-01
Albert Complex
Singapore 189969

Canada
Nelson/Thomson Learning
1120 Birchmount Road
Scarborough, Ontario M1K 5G4
Canada

Library of Congress Cataloging-in-Publication Data
Cohen, Robert, 1941–
   Chiseled in sand: perspectives on change in human services orga-
nizations/Robert Cohen, Jessye Cohen.
      p.   cm.
   Includes bibliographical references (p. 285) and index.
   ISBN 0-534-36485-3 (hc.)
      1. Human services—United States—Management.
2. Organizational change—United States. 3. Human services—
Management. I. Title.
HV91.C593   1999
658.3—dc21   99-37930

♻ This book is printed on acid-free recycled paper.

For Sid Oglesby, Dianne Apter, Paula Trief, Joe Himmelsbach, Bob Sprafkin, and the memory of Steve Apter, early travelers on the challenging course of change.

∼ R.C.

For my mother, Nancy and my brothers, Nick and Tim.

∼ J.C.

CONTENTS

PREFACE

This book grew out of a keen interest in the profound changes occurring in the field of human services. Much has been written about *what* these changes are: the emerging focus on providing holistic services tailored to each individual's needs and strengths; the importance of taking into account the context in which a person lives—family, community, and culture; and the reconceptualization of the relationship between providers and recipients of services, based on the desire to empower both parties. These changes, as well as others in the field of human services, parallel trends within the broader society.

While there is still a pressing need to enhance our understanding of these emerging trends, in this volume our primary focus is the *process* rather than the *content* of these changes. We are interested in *how* persons can bring about innovative change as well as *how* individuals can more effectively cope with the uncertainty and stress that accompany change. Given the rapid pace at which change is occurring and the enormous impact it is having on individuals—both providers and consumers—as well as human services organizations and institutions, we believe that more attention should be given to the change process.

The business sector has been inundated by theoretical and practical writings on personal and organizational approaches to change. Some of this material, which is cited in Chapters 1 and 2, has considerable relevance to human services. On the whole, however, the field of human services has suffered from a paucity of information on how to effectively design, implement, and manage the changes that have become a routine and integral part of this field.

Although we have provided a brief conceptual overview of the change process, our primary goal is to share with the reader actual examples of how change occurs or is coped with in a variety of human services settings. In many cases we, the authors, have been directly involved in the change processes described. While most of the case narratives focus on mental health issues, the concepts and dynamics of change are applicable to all human services settings.

We believe that this book will be of interest to a wide audience and can be used in a variety of human services settings. Our book is intended to complement more theoretical textbooks in a variety of graduate and undergraduate courses. We made an effort to present the material in an easy-to-read, accessible format. By providing students and teachers with a series of case narratives and other firsthand accounts, we hope to enhance understanding of how change actually occurs in the field and to assist in integrating theory and practice in mental health and other human services. While the book has direct applicability for courses in community mental health, social work, nursing, mental health and health administration, community and organizational psychology, and management of not-for-profit organizations, it also has relevance for all undergraduate and graduate professional training for human services. While the primary target audience is students, the book may also be useful for professionals in the human services who are trying to cope with a rapidly changing environment. Lay persons interested in understanding how change is affecting mental health and other human services also may find this book of interest.

ACKNOWLEDGMENTS

We owe great thanks to all of the people who helped to make this book possible. First and foremost, we would both like to thank Carol Ishler for all of her hard work and time. In addition to patiently and competently preparing the manuscript, she consistently provided encouragement and support throughout this project. We express our appreciation to Jeri Baker, Research Associate and Family Advocate, who authored the chapter on parents' perspectives on their children's services systems, and we are grateful to all the parents who participated in the interview process. We also thank all of the young people who agreed to participate in interviews about their experiences in human services: Abby, Anne, Jessica, Judith, Daniel, Erin, and Pat. Lisa Gebo and the staff of Brooks/Cole provided useful feedback and assistance at all stages of development, and we are appreciative of their willingness to support this project. We also thank the reviewers for their constructive criticism and suggestions.

Others deserve credit for listening to our constant dialogues and monologues about "the book." Both of us are grateful to Nancy, Tim, and Nick Cohen for putting up with us and our worries, frustrations, and creative ruminations during the writing of this book.

Each of us also wants to thank some persons who have been particularly supportive.

JC: I want to thank Jennifer Anderson, Zoë Kafatou, Erin Murphy, Victoria Pearson, and Marissa Walsh for their patience and support. I owe a debt of gratitude to the teachers, both formal and informal, who made me believe that this work was worth pursuing and helped me find the beginning of the path.

RC: I especially want to acknowledge the following people at the Virginia Treatment Center for Children and the Department of Psychiatry of Virginia Commonwealth University: Isaac Abraham, Jeri Baker, John Blatecky, Frank Boon, Debbie Cole, Nancy Doyle, Pat Doyle, Frances Dyson, Corliss Hanson, Jeri Hosick, Jim Levenson, Barbara Nobles, Donald Oswald, Barbara Ozlin, Dean Parmelee, Joel Silverman, Nirbhay Singh, Ron Snead, Neil Sonenklar, Bela Sood, and Shirley Wiley. They have been good companions on this tumultuous journey of change.

INTRODUCTION

The process of writing this book may be viewed as a metaphor for functioning within the current human services environment. Coming from a traditional relationship—father and daughter—we had to confront a number of difficult challenges as we strove to redefine our roles in our new partnership as coauthors of this book.

At times we were able to identify and mobilize our complementary perspectives and skills successfully. For instance, the differences in our experience within the field allowed us to provide diverse and occasionally contrasting perspectives. In addition to occupying different roles, that is, administrator/teacher versus resource development specialist, the nature and timing of our training and experience also affected our views. For instance, viewing current human services situations through the eyes of someone who has been trained and worked in more traditional approaches is not the same as viewing them from the perspective of someone who has grown up in the current climate and has no other experiential frame of reference.

Although our different perspectives often served as assets, we occasionally experienced conflict, making it difficult at times to perform our functions as writing partners. Fortunately, through persistence and good communication, we successfully negotiated our differences and performed new roles in order to achieve our mutual goal: to complete this book. In many ways our efforts to redefine roles and enter into a different type of relationship mirrors current trends. Individuals and organizations who previously functioned independently and sometimes in competition with each other are now coming together to form productive, mutually beneficial partnerships.

THE ROOTS OF OUR VIEWS

Each of us became interested in the issue of how human services systems function through different, though admittedly connected, routes. By sharing our formative experiences, we hope to accomplish several purposes. These examples illustrate some of the dynamics that occur within human services organizations and systems. In addition to highlighting some of the forces that influence organizational practice, these examples also underscore a few of the problems that precipitated the current reform initiatives within human services. By presenting experiences that contributed to our appreciation and understanding, we hope to impart to readers a sense of our individual orientations and biases.

R.C.: My first insight into organizational dynamics occurred while I was attending graduate school in the 1960s in a small northern city. At that time, I became involved in a number of civil rights activities at the university and in the surrounding community. It did not take me long to realize that institutions, as well as other organizational entities, operated according to a set of rules that were different from the lessons I had learned in my high school civics class. With my incomplete education, I was not prepared for the intriguing and sometimes puzzling dynamics of organizational behavior I encountered. In time, I would learn to understand some of the fundamental principles and forces that shaped the way in which agencies and institutions made decisions, performed their functions, and interacted with other organizational entities, but at the time I had difficulty making sense of many of my experiences within organizational settings. Following are a few of the incidents that heightened my awareness of the unique rules of logic that govern organizational behavior.

• In 1963, the local civil rights group mounted a petition campaign to gather support for the voter rights initiative in the South. Hoping to increase the visibility of our efforts, several of us approached the mayor of the city and asked him to sign our petition. To our surprise, he neither agreed nor declined to sign the petition based on his beliefs about the cause. Instead, he inquired about who else had signed the petition and suggested that we acquire the signatures of other prominent individuals before asking for his support. His reluctance to sign what appeared to be a relatively innocuous statement in this urban northern environment surprised me at the time. This was one of my first lessons in the importance of context in the decision-making process. Who is in favor of, or opposed to, a particular position or action and how one's stance on the issue is perceived by others are often more critical to decision makers than the substance and merit of the issue.

• During my graduate training in clinical psychology, I participated in a practicum in a large Veterans Administration neuropsychiatric hospital. Once a week a diagnostic conference was held in which patients were assessed for the purpose of establishing a formal diagnosis. After attending these conferences for a while, I observed a curious phenomenon. Occasionally a patient's current symptoms and functioning were discrepant with a previous diagnostic label that had been given to the patient. Invariably the attending psychiatrist decided to use the previously established diagnosis rather than to revise it in accordance with the patient's current behavior. When I asked one of the psychiatrists why the historical diagnosis always prevailed, he looked at me quizzically and explained, "Of course we would not want to alter the diagnosis because it might negatively impact the patient's disability benefits." While the motivation for this rationale at first glance appeared to be altruistic, though not rational, upon reflection another possibility emerged. Could it be that changing the diagnosis would necessitate additional effort and paperwork, while keeping the same diagnosis required placing a checkmark in the box on the assessment form marked "no change since last diagnosis"? My naive mind began to grasp a fundamental principle of institutional behavior: The path of least resistance is almost always the most desirable path.

• For nearly a full academic year, the university community struggled with the question of whether it should compete with athletic teams from other universities that maintained a policy of racial segregation. One faction of the campus believed that the best opportunity for influencing the policy of these other institutions of higher education was to participate on a playing field with black students from opposing schools. Another segment thought that segregation was morally wrong and that we were not only condoning this practice but also contributing to its perpetuation through a financial agreement that called for ticket proceeds to be shared by both schools. After considerable debate and protest, the chancellor delegated the decision to the university athletic board, which was responsible for overseeing the sports program. The board's decision to continue competing with the segregated schools was reported in the campus newspaper. The board's chair explained that the board had wrestled with the many facets of this issue and had concluded that maintaining involvement with these schools would keep the channels of communication open and, therefore, enable the university to influence the segregated schools toward a policy of integration.

The next day, to my surprise, the campus newspaper printed a statement by the chancellor congratulating the athletic board for having the wisdom to decide to terminate athletic competition with segregated universities. When I asked a university official to reconcile the discrepancy between the published report of the board's decision to continue athletic competition with segregated schools and the chancellor's laudatory statement on the board's position to discontinue athletic relationships with these universities, I received another valuable lesson in organizational dynamics. In order to reconcile the apparent contradiction between the two statements, the university administrator drew an analogy between the chancellor's behavior and the Supreme Court. He explained that while the court, or in this instance the athletic board, was responsible for issuing a ruling based on the evidence, it was the duty of the chief justice—in this case, the chancellor—to interpret the meaning of this ruling. Therefore, according to the university official to whom I spoke, the chancellor was simply translating what the athletic board's statement actually meant. The university would no longer engage in athletic competition with segregated schools.

The analogy between the Chief Justice of the Supreme Court and the chancellor struck me as odd at the time and, even today, offends my sense of logic. This incident, however, provided me with insight into how major conflicts within or between organizations are resolved in a manner that allows the unsuccessful faction to save face. With mounting pressure from the university community to discontinue the support of segregated institutions, the chancellor wanted to change the existing policy. Yet he did not want to usurp the athletic board's governance role. By "interpreting" or, in today's political parlance, "putting a spin" on the board's statement, the chancellor was able to successfully change the university's policy on playing segregated schools without publicly criticizing the athletic board.

These episodes, as well as others I experienced during my graduate student years, forced me to reassess my basic assumptions about organizational behavior. I began to understand that the basic rules of organizational logic that we learned as children do not always apply. An agency's course of action is more frequently driven by self-preservation than by its stated missions and goals. Political and economic forces have greater influence than programmatic philosophy. The hidden agenda is often more powerful than the stated plan.

J.C.: One of the strongest forces that influenced my decision to become involved in human services work was my own experience as a consumer of mental health services. As a consumer I felt a lack of advocacy on behalf of those with mental health needs. Fortunately, I was educated in the mental health field and was able to be my own advocate. However, I recognized a dire need for others to have this resource to draw upon since navigating the field of service providers and services is a difficult task for individuals in need. A few examples from my own experience illustrate the need for more information and resources.

I have struggled with depression throughout my life. During my first year of college I had a particularly difficult time managing my depression and being in school. My provider was in Virginia and I was in school in Massachusetts. I tried to continue treatment with the doctor in Virginia, but it proved difficult to reach him by telephone, and he was unable to evaluate me from such a distance. I went to the college mental health services several times, but I found them lacking and not very helpful. Furthermore, the mental health services at the college were designed to address short-term crises, so staff were unprepared to offer services beyond three or four sessions. A family friend recommended a psychiatrist in my college town. I made an appointment with him, desperately hoping he would be able to help me.

During our first visit I felt okay about the discussion. This was the first time I would be seeing the same provider for medication and therapy. Most of our discussion focused on my history. He decided to lower my medication and add two other drugs. I was a little concerned that he seemed to be relying heavily on the *DSM-IV* (*Diagnostic and Statistical Manual of Mental Disorders*) on his desk, but I dismissed this concern. During my second session, he continued to respond to my descriptions by looking up each "symptom" in the manual.

We began to discuss some of the other aspects of my life. When he asked me about my relationships, I explained to him that I was dating another woman. He responded by suggesting that perhaps I was depressed because I was involved in a "socially unacceptable lesbian relationship." I was shocked and disappointed that he was not the beacon I had hoped to find. More importantly, this man worked in a town with a significant lesbian population. Undoubtedly he was sharing his "clinical opinion" with other women who came to see him. His diagnosis had been hasty and inaccurate, and I terminated treatment.

As a footnote to my experience with the college health service, I returned there some months later and explained to the staff psychologist what had happened with the psychiatrist in town. She seemed surprised and said, "He's very good. We refer students to his office all the time." She agreed that he might be overzealous about the use of medication, but she did not seem to take any of my concerns seriously.

This experience left me feeling discouraged and disempowered. As a young consumer, I felt as if this mental health services system was not designed to meet my needs at all. I decided at that point that I would devote some of my energy and time to fighting such irresponsibility and educating people about their roles as consumers.

Most of this effort has been informal. I talk about my own experience as a consumer so that other people will break the silence, too. In our culture we talk about physical health with relative ease, though there are certainly complications, but we shroud mental health issues in shame, embarrassment, and silence. It is important to talk about the things that make us uncomfortable. As a lesbian and as a mental health services consumer, I deserve to know my rights and demand the care I need. We must have a forum for this education and a vocabulary with which to discuss these issues.

My experience of organizational dynamics began long before I was aware of their complexity. Beyond my personal experience as a consumer, I have always had an interest in being an advocate and working to help other people. From a young age I believed it was my responsibility to volunteer some of my time to help make the world a better place, an idealism that has been tempered but not forgotten. In college I spent a great deal of time in discussions about creating community and how to maintain mutual respect and comfort. So many meetings of organizations were bogged down with bureaucracy and process that it was often difficult to reach the goal of the meeting.

My contribution to this book brings a younger perspective to the discussion of change in human services. I present my own narrative account of and the lessons I learned from working in a nonprofit organization. I also drew upon the experience of some of my peers to write a chapter based on interviews with young people who have worked in human services. Clearly the senior author of this book has far more experience working in the field, so his case narratives make up the majority of the text. We have collaborated in creating the learning tools and the structure of the text, and we both participated in the research on organizational behavior.

One might ask what is so special about these insights? Only a naive individual would be surprised by the conclusion that factors other than altruism and logic play a significant role in influencing how individuals and organizations behave. It is not, however, the basic tenets of organizational dynamics that require further education; it is the manner in which agencies and institutions enact these principles in the course of responding to opportunities and threats that presents a challenge to those of us involved in understanding and working with organizations. Knowing that political forces influence decisions made by human services agencies is not the same as understanding how the players in an organizational scenario identify what they want to accomplish, develop strategies to achieve their established objectives, and interact with each other for the purpose of negotiating their individual interests and common purposes. What is fascinating about organizational function, from our perspective, are the intricate details of how complex elements in an organizational system respond to perceived opportunities and threats. We have been particularly interested in the dynamics of change: How do individuals and groups in the human services attempt to make services more responsive to the needs of individuals, families, and communities? How do competing political, social, and economic forces interact to produce change? How do agencies and systems adapt to changes that are imposed on them, and what are the courses of organizational adaptation and resistance? What strategies can an individual use to facilitate constructive change and assist organizations to adapt to externally imposed changes?

We have struggled with these questions throughout our careers. Occasionally, we have felt the momentary satisfaction of clearly understanding a complex situation or successfully executing an organizational change strategy. Most of the time, however, we plod along, tending to the countless details accompanying the organizational change process, fending off crises that distract us from our desired course of action, and trying to steal a few minutes to reflect on what is happening and what needs to be done to achieve our goals. In recent years the pace of change has accelerated. As we try to keep up with the rapid flow of events, it becomes important, if not essential, to maintain a systems perspective that allows us to understand what is happening in the environment and how we might act to constructively influence the change process.

In this book we chronicle some of the experiences and observations we have had in our struggle to understand and influence the change process in a variety of human services settings. Our paths have been neither conventional nor linear. We have worked in academic and applied settings, spending time in small community organizations, large bureaucracies, and highly structured institutions. The diversity of our work experiences has probably been both a liability and an asset. Having experience in such a diverse array of human services settings has allowed us to identify not only the differences among these environments but also the similarities. Communication may be easier in a small single-site agency than in a large state agency spread out over multiple divisions and geographic settings. The people who work in these organizations, however, share a common interest in wanting to know what is expected of them, feeling good about providing services that actually help people, and being anxious about impending changes.

It is important to us to acknowledge the concerns we have not addressed thoroughly. We recognize that since most of the book is drawn from our own experiences, our representation of people in human services is limited. Though we discuss race, class, gender, and sexual orientation to some extent, we know that our own experiences do not encompass the concerns of all people involved in human services. With unlimited space and time, we would have presented a broader perspective. A crucial point arises from this discussion: No matter how many general trends we can identify, the experience of each individual in a human services organization will be drastically different from that of his or her colleagues.

There are certain areas of human services that we have not addressed. We have not covered the justice system, many aspects of health care, and other important service areas such as housing and transportation. We also have not focused on many of the important approaches to changing human services that are initiated outside of the established hierarchy, for example, consumer advocacy and community organizations.

Our goal has been to present our own experiences as examples and to pose questions that allow readers to consider issues related to their own interests. It has not been our intention to provide readers with a cookbook on how to create and cope with change. Recipes may be useful for baking delicious cakes, but we have not found one that is helpful in making a human services agency more responsive to the people it serves. If one wants to foster constructive change within an organizational setting, it is necessary to have a sound perspective on the change process, a good understanding of the specific situation, and sufficient sensitivity to the potential impact of the various forces in the environment. With this conceptual framework, it is possible to know what can be accomplished using change management tools such as strategic planning and communication skills. Equally important, a good perspective enables us all to know what we cannot accomplish.

In the pages that follow, we expose readers to the process of change within a variety of human services settings. In conjunction with describing actual events and situations, we offer a personal and admittedly subjective set of observations on the forces and factors that have facilitated and impeded these change processes and have helped the individuals involved to adapt to these changes when they have occurred.

HOW THIS BOOK IS ORGANIZED

As already stated, this book has the unique quality of being a collaborative effort of two authors with very different perspectives. We are a father and daughter team, representing years of experience in a variety of human services settings, on the one hand, and a fairly recent college graduate's perspective on the other. We have combined the strengths of these differences in perspective to create a text that addresses a multitude of issues in human services now and for the past thirty years.

Our narrative styles and the variety of learning tools we use encourage students to get very close to our own experiences and to think about their future experiences in these fields. We have incorporated contemporary organizational theory and relevant historical information into the first section of the book to provide a theoretical framework for the rest of the book. This text explores many topics relevant to the work in a variety of courses and is reader friendly.

In Section I we provide a conceptual framework for organizational change. We discuss the forces that influence change in the first chapter. In Chapter 2 we present a theoretical perspective on organizational development and describe current and recent trends of thought in this area.

In Section II we look at change from the perspectives of organizations. We present two chapters that focus on dramatic change in a children's psychiatric hospital. Another chapter discusses the development of a system of family-centered services. The final chapter in this section is an account of a young person's first experience working in a human services organization.

In Section III we present change from a systems perspective, including the experience of working in a large state government agency and participating in the creation and implementation of a statewide system of children's services. This section also includes a chapter on the issues encountered in evaluating an innovative approach to community policing and a description of how a statewide system of children's services attempted, in a rational and constructive manner, to address concerns about appropriateness, quality, and cost of services .

In Section IV we present unique perspectives from the field. We include a narrative chapter exploring children's services in another country. This section includes two chapters based on interviews. The first interview chapter focuses on parents navigating the children's services system on behalf of their children. The second interview chapter presents the perspectives of young human services workers. We also explore the directions in which we believe human services are heading.

Learning Devices

Case Examples   We have written a series of narrative chapters describing experiences that we have had working in human services in a variety of settings. These provide students with a thorough depiction of each situation and a context for the organizational theory that we present early in the book.

Interviews   We have included two chapters based on interviews: one from the perspectives of consumers and the other from the perspectives of young workers in human services. These chapters add to the human element of the text. The chapter focusing on young workers will be of particular interest to students because most of the individuals speaking are recent college graduates.

Points to Ponder   At the conclusion of each chapter, we include a list of questions to encourage further discussion of the topics raised in this chapter. The instructor may use these questions in class or ask students to discuss them with each other. The questions require that students consider the conceptual framework of each chapter, as well as the narrative.

From Classroom to Community   At the end of each chapter we provide a scenario that involves the use of one or more lessons from the preceding chapter. Students are asked to imagine themselves in a certain situation that could arise during work in human services or to study the dynamics of change in an actual human services organization. Our hope is that these scenarios will engage students in thinking about their own roles as potential workers in human services. It is the first step in applying the concepts of change from classroom learning to outside experience.

UNDERSTANDING CHANGE IN THE HUMAN SERVICES: A CONCEPTUAL FRAMEWORK

CHAPTER 1

CHANGE
Why All the Commotion?

*There is no reason anyone would want a computer in
their home.*

~ Ken Olsen, President, Chairman, and Founder, Digital
Equipment Corporation, 1977

T he problems and challenges currently encountered by human services
consumers, workers, and organizations are not unique to this field. All
segments of society—families, businesses, governments, and a host of other
social institutions—are experiencing rapid and profound changes. If we
wish to understand why these changes are occurring and how we can deal
more effectively with them, it is necessary to understand the broader picture and to be aware of the forces that are driving change. In this chapter
we discuss some of the political, economic, technological, cultural, social,
and programmatic forces that are impacting human services entities and
present some of the strategies for change.

~

In her remarkable book *Within Our Reach: Breaking the Cycle of Disadvantage,* Lisbeth Schorr (1988) reports the results of her nationwide search to
identify programs that have successfully addressed the needs of disadvan-

taged children and families. She describes more than twenty exemplary health and human services programs that demonstrated improved outcomes among children in disadvantaged families, including reductions in rates of school dropout, arrest for violent crime, teenage pregnancy, and welfare dependence. Five years later, nearly half of the programs she cites had gone out of business (Schorr, 1994).

The dramatic failure rate among these exemplary ventures is disturbing. In spite of their apparent effectiveness in serving children and families, a significant number of these successful programs were unable to sustain their viability. Schorr (1994) indicates that part of the reason for the high failure rate is that the systems within which these programs function are not designed to support comprehensive, flexible approaches to meeting individual needs within the context of the family and community. Conventional methods of financing, regulating, managing, and holding programs accountable actually undermine the innovative approaches employed by these programs.

The high mortality rate of these exemplary programs provides a sobering reminder of the vulnerability and complexity of human services programs. It is not sufficient simply to have good intentions and a clear idea of what children and families need. Nor is it adequate to have well-trained employees equipped with an array of conceptually and empirically sound program strategies. It is also essential to understand the context in which programs operate and to be prepared to cope with the financial, organizational, and political dynamics of the entities in the surrounding environment that support and control service programs. This challenge is difficult under stable conditions. If one adds into the mix the rapid pace of change that we are experiencing in all aspects of modern life, the challenge becomes truly daunting.

Everywhere we turn the accelerating rate of change is evident. The demographic profile of the population has changed significantly. Persons over age sixty-five comprise approximately 13 percent of the population and the most rapidly growing age group in this country. In 1950, three-quarters of households were married; today, fewer than one-quarter are. The percentage of women between ages twenty-five and fifty-four in the workforce has increased more than 125 percent in the past forty years. More than 50 percent of the workforce expansion between 1986 and the year 2000 came from minority groups (Fosler, 1990). Between 1978 and 1995 young workers changed jobs an average of nine times between the ages of eighteen and thirty-two (U.S. Bureau of Labor Statistics, 1998). The type of work that people are engaged in has also changed dramatically. In the early part of the twentieth century there was a shift from agriculture to manufacturing. Recently, the service industry has replaced manufacturing as the major source of employment in the United States. In 1992, 71 percent of all workers were employed in service-related occupations while 26 percent were employed in manufacturing and only 3 percent in agriculture (U.S. Bureau of the Census, 1993, Table 644).

The dramatic changes that have occurred during the past several decades have impacted individuals and families served by human services programs, persons who work for human services agencies, and the manner in which services are provided. Given the likelihood that change will continue to occur at a similar or accelerated pace in the foreseeable future, consumers, workers, and the service delivery system will continue to be impacted. If we are to understand how changes affect various aspects of the human services system, we must be aware of the forces that are driving change. Even more important, if we wish to learn how to cope with these changes, we must not only be aware of these forces but also must understand how to develop strategies that enable us to respond in ways that improve our ability to meet the needs and support the strengths of individuals and families served by the system.

While some changes have been instigated from within the human services environment, it is evident that many changes are being driven by broader societal pressures and sources outside of the human services community. Students, practitioners, and administrators involved in human services need to understand the rationale, content, and strategies associated with their specific service programs. If education is limited to the internal operation of human services, service providers may not be adequately prepared to deal with the challenges that confront them. Service providers also should have an appreciation of the forces that shape change and the approaches that can be utilized to guide these forces constructively. Personnel also need to develop perspectives and skills to cope with the unrelenting, rapid pace of change that pervades the human services.

FORCES THAT IMPACT HUMAN SERVICES ORGANIZATIONS

Factors that influence organizational function can be classified according to the nature of the force as well as its point of origin. The most common types of such forces are political, economic, technological, social, cultural, and programmatic. These factors may originate inside or outside the organization and, therefore, may be classified as emanating from the internal or external environment.

What are some of the major factors influencing change in human services organizations? To adequately address this question, it is necessary to understand the historical context of human services organizations as well as the specific forces that are currently affecting these organizations. Consider the following:

Political Influences

The fact that political forces influence organizational functioning probably does not surprise anyone. At the most basic level, the programmatic direction of agencies operated or funded by government entities is determined largely by the political philosophy and priorities of incumbent elected officials.

For example, if the governor of a state perceives that his or her political support comes from constituents who are concerned about the safety of their communities, the priorities for state agencies are likely to reflect this concern. In this scenario, correctional facilities are likely to add new beds, mental health agencies may place greater emphasis on serving individuals in institutional rather than community settings, and support for homeless people may be limited to initiatives that decrease their visibility in middle- and upper-class neighborhoods. While there may be consensus that the level of violence in communities is unacceptable, it is unlikely that much energy will be directed at gun control. Under a conservative political administration, protecting an individual's right to bear arms will be considered more important than reducing access to instruments of aggression. Conversely, a liberal administration confronted with increased violence in schools will probably promote programs that deal with environmental conditions that spawn aggression but will not be likely to support initiatives that permanently remove aggressors from the school environment. In this latter instance, the decision to intervene at the community level rather than banish perpetrators—particularly younger individuals—to institutional settings may be driven more by political belief than scientific evidence. The liberal perspective that society's problems are caused by environmental deficiencies is based largely on a political philosophy rather than an abundance of empirical data supporting the efficacy of community-based interventions.

Political forces also influence human services policy and practice through intergovernmental dynamics. Each level of government—federal, state, or local—contends that it is in a unique position to best respond to the needs of consumers of human services. City and county officials claim that their understanding of local conditions places them in the best position to make decisions about how to allocate resources to human services programs. Federal officials, citing constitutional provisions and other federal statutes, justify their role as essential to ensuring the rights of those in need of services. Legislators and administrators at the state level assert their expertise and knowledge of local needs and defend their role in ensuring equitable provision of services to all citizens in their domain. State representatives typically portray the federal government as attempting to build a larger bureaucracy by meddling in local affairs. At the same time, state officials justify their involvement by adopting the federal role of ensuring equal access to services for all citizens of the state.

The interaction among these governmental entities often has a profound effect on the shape and scope of human services. The initial design of a statewide initiative to improve services for a specific population may be based primarily on the research and best practices in that field. Even if this design has been demonstrated to be effective, it is unlikely to be adopted unless it can be modified to be compatible with local conditions as well as the requirements of federal agencies. The Comprehensive Services Act for At Risk Youth and Families, Virginia's statewide initiative for children with serious emotional and behavioral disorders (see Chapters 9 and 10) illustrates this dynamic. Rather than adopting a "one-size-fits-all" program model, state officials promulgated a general set of service principles that emphasized child- and family-oriented services delivered within community settings. Each locality was expected to develop a service system based on these principles that was responsive to the needs and conditions of that community. By promoting local choice, the architects of this initiative encouraged local ownership and empowerment. Equally important, they were able to overcome the objections of local officials and gain needed support for passage of this legislation. On the other hand, the absence of specific directions for localities increased the likelihood that service programs would not be implemented according to their original design. This tradeoff illustrates the interplay between program philosophy and intergovernmental conflict. Whether or not this program initiative will ultimately be more effective because it allows for local flexibility is an empirical question that can only be answered through experience. What is certain is that the interplay among various levels of government has had a profound effect on shaping this initiative.

Using mental health services as an example, we can demonstrate the relationship between political forces and mental health approaches by comparing the 1950s and the 1960s. In the 1950s, the United States adopted a conservative, isolationist position, possibly in response to the trauma and turmoil of World War II. During that period, the two major mental health modalities were psychoanalysis, with its emphasis on unconscious motivation and realignment of the individual psyche, and the placement of persons with mental health problems in large, remote, public psychiatric institutions, a trend that reached its peak in the 1950s with more than a half million people residing in state institutions throughout the country (Lamb and Associates, 1976).

In comparison, consider the social activism of the 1960s: the civil rights movement, the war against poverty, the Vietnam protest, and the initial emergence of the women's movement. The politically liberal climate and the willingness to spend money on social programs was accompanied by a philosophy of mental health services that targeted environmental factors as causes of agents of dysfunctional behavior. The birth of the community mental health movement, with its initial focus on strengthening communities in order to enhance mental health functioning, and the emergence of behavior modification approaches that linked individuals' behavior to the reinforcement received from the environment occurred during the 1960s and may be viewed as direct support for the correlation between political ideology and theories of human behavior (Levine and Levine, 1970).

In addition to being affected by the prevailing political orientation, human services organizations are also impacted by specific political decisions. For example, in New York State, family members, professionals, and human services agencies had been seeking programmatic and fiscal support for family-oriented services for many years without much success. During the 1982 gubernatorial campaign, Mario Cuomo successfully used the metaphor of New York State as a family to propel himself to an upset victory. Shortly after the election, his aides developed a multimillion-dollar budget proposal for family-oriented initiatives in the human services, hoping to capitalize on his campaign slogan. As a result of this budget submission, funding was appropriated for a number of significant family services and support programs that had previously been proposed but rejected.

Human services professionals, particularly those in academic settings, often disparage the role of political forces in shaping policy and practice. They believe that compassion and rational analysis ought to be the sole factors that guide policy decisions. An alternative view about the role of politics in policy formulation (Stone, 1997) suggests that objective principles and rational analysis will never be sufficient for explaining or predicting human behavior. Stone asserts that we are political creatures in our daily lives as well as in governance and urges us to accept and incorporate politics as an essential component of our analytical activities. She states that analytical concepts, problem statements, and policy instruments should be recognized as political claims instead of as universal truths. Toward this end, she favors the model of society as a political community rather than a market.

The Impact of Economics

The amount of money a human services organization receives is dependent on a number of factors. The general state of the economy obviously has an impact. In times of economic prosperity, both governmental allocation and philanthropic donations are likely to be higher. The relationship between the health of the economy and the availability of funding is not always linear. In times of crisis, such as natural disasters and high unemployment, government may choose to allocate greater sums of money to help those in need. In these instances, as well as others, political priorities may take precedence over economic indicators in determining the funding allocation for a human services initiative.

In addition to the amount of money an organization receives, the source and purpose of funding may also affect human services programs and organizations. A community may be more likely to initiate an innovative program that is supported by a state or federal demonstration project or foundation grant than to allocate dollars from its scarce pool of local resources. Yet a program supported by time-limited outside funds is less likely to endure than one that is financially as well as programmatically supported by the local community.

The nature of the funding mechanism also has an impact on how an organization provides services. If a funding agency chooses to provide financial support for children's services by calculating the actual cost of each service program, service providers will be more inclined to offer expensive residential services rather than nonresidential services that cost less. However, if a funding agency wants to accomplish the programmatic objective of encouraging the development of nonresidential, community-based services, financial incentives and disincentives may be incorporated into the funding formula to reinforce desired programmatic outcomes. If an agency knows that it does not have to pay anything to place a child in a state-operated residential program, it is more likely to choose the residential placement. Conversely, if a county social services department knows that it will have to contribute a higher proportion of local share for residential services or is required to pay a financial penalty for exceeding its quota of residential placements, it will be more reluctant to purchase residential services.

Historically, government and not-for-profit mental health and other human services organizations have not been concerned with the nature of funding mechanisms. Many services either have been subsidized or paid for on a contractual basis. Thus, the relationship between the manner in which funding is allocated and how services are delivered has not received much attention. As mentioned, cost-based funding encourages service expansion since the amount of funding received is dependent on the quantity of services delivered.

In recent years, with the increased emphasis on accountability and fiscal constraint, more sophisticated methods of funding have been introduced in the fields of mental health and other human services. In some instances, capitation methodologies have been applied. In such approaches, a provider receives a fixed amount of funding for an individual or a population. The provider is responsible for providing all services required to meet the client's needs. If the actual cost of the services is less than the capitated rate, the provider may retain the surplus. If services cost more than the amount allocated under the capitation arrangement, the provider is responsible for absorbing the additional expenses.

At one level, this fiscal mechanism encourages the use of preventive, community-based service modalities that are typically less expensive than as well as compatible with an early-intervention, less restrictive service philosophy. However, the capitation funding methodology also presents potential problems. A provider may be encouraged to offer fewer services in order to save money unless there are safeguards to ensure that services appropriate to an individual's needs are provided. Fortunately, a variety of accountability methods can be used to ensure appropriate provision of services. Such methods include eliciting feedback from consumers, requiring agencies to provide periodic reports on performance, and auditing agency records to verify compliance.

Also in recent years, increased emphasis has been placed on outcome-based performance (Bickman and Rog, 1998; Kane, 1997; Lyons et al., 1997). Although outcome-oriented approaches have been discussed more frequently than they have been implemented, the notion of linking payment with achievement of specific and mutually agreed upon results has considerable appeal as a means of aligning fiscal incentives with program objectives.

Technological Advances

From a programmatic perspective, mental health services have been enhanced by new technology. The proliferation of psychopharmacological research has made it possible to treat many people more effectively with fewer side effects (Lader and Herrington, 1996; Parmelee, 1996). The development of more sophisticated behavioral therapies has provided consumers with alternative ways to cope with stress and has allowed individuals with serious behavioral problems to be treated in less restrictive settings (O'Donohue and Krasner, 1995; Singh, 1997). While the alternatives available to mental health consumers and practitioners are still limited, genetic, biochemical, and psychosocial research continues to proliferate. The findings from these investigations are likely to have a profound impact on how mental health and other human services are provided in the twenty-first century.

Other technological progress, most notably advances in information processing and communication, appear to be having a mixed impact on human services. While consumers, providers, and policy makers have greater access to data that will aid them in making decisions about services, these technologies also create unintended problems for consumers and practitioners. For example, in an effort to increase efficiency, many service organizations have introduced complex menu-driven telephone answering systems. These devices may yield financial savings through the reduction of clerical personnel, but the frustration of attempting to work through the maze of digital options does little to enhance a consumer's view of these systems as person centered or customer oriented.

The accelerated speed at which communication occurs through various apparatus, such as computers and fax machines, also has produced some deleterious consequences. Increased expectations of productivity—as well as the added burden of having to respond to e-mail, voice mail, fax correspondence, and other information-processing devices—generate stress and do not contribute to the mental well-being of those individuals required to keep up with the dizzying array of communication alternatives.

Social and Cultural Changes

As mainstream America becomes less homogenous, human services agencies have been forced to reexamine the manner in which services are provided. Spokespersons for ethnic minority groups, which are growing in size and strength, have effectively communicated that these populations historically have been underserved. In addition to receiving too few services, the services that have been delivered are often not responsive to the cultural norms of clients. Changes in gender role and status are also having a significant impact on the planning, organization, and delivery of human services. The women's movement has dramatically changed the role of women in the workplace, as well as the dynamics of contemporary families. As consumers, women are asserting that providers pay more attention to their unique needs. While women have always played a critical role as providers of human services, traditionally they have been underrepresented in positions of authority and power. This imbalance seems to be shifting as more women assume leadership positions in human services organizations.

The increased visibility of sexual minorities has also influenced mental health and other human services sectors. Although consensus is not close at hand, the fact that there are fewer depictions of homosexuality as mental illness or as unnatural and sinful behavior signals a shift in attitude toward gays and lesbians.

There is growing recognition that a single approach to providing services is not sufficient to respond to the wide array of groups that seek assistance. Providing culturally compatible services with a workforce that is demographically compatible and culturally and socially attuned to the diverse range of consumers seeking services presents a formidable challenge to administrators at all levels. In an effort to be responsive to demands for cultural competence, program managers have sometimes rushed to fill service positions with persons who look and talk like their clients without giving sufficient attention to whether such persons possess the skills necessary to respond to clients' needs. Good listening skills and the ability to be empathic may be more important requisites for providing culturally competent services than simply matching consumers and providers according to identifiable demographic, social, and cultural indicators.

The influence of new cultural values has created dilemmas for all organizations in both Western and Eastern cultures (Kao, Sinha, and Sek-Hong, 1995). In response to Japan's successes in enhancing productivity, many U.S. organizations have adopted management approaches that emphasize teamwork and common purpose. These approaches fly in the face of the cultural emphasis placed on individualism in the United States. Conversely, the Eastern values of collectivism and loyalty to culture appear to be breaking down. This shift has created interesting and difficult dilemmas for Eastern organizations forced to confront the erosion of paternalism and organizational trust as manifested by the growing role of trade unions in oriental organizations.

While there has been some emphasis on teamwork in mental health and other human services—such as milieu therapy and interdisciplinary teams—much of the activity in these fields has been conducted by solo practitioners or professionals functioning in a clearly hierarchical structure. Incorporating genuine teamwork into human services organizational structures requires considerable ingenuity and adaptation on the part of administrators and practitioners.

The increased recognition of the uniqueness and rights of multiple cultural and ethnic groups has been accompanied by an emerging emphasis on consumer empowerment and satisfaction. Mental health groups such as the National Alliance for the Mentally Ill and the Mental Health Consumers Association have shifted the balance of power away from the professionals who previously dominated the field. In addition to demonstrating their ability to produce tangible results in the form of legislative changes and increased financial support, these advocacy groups have actively encouraged providers to be more responsive to the needs of consumers and members of their families (Levine and Perkins, 1997). This trend is consistent with the themes of common purpose and teamwork being promoted in modern Western organizations. The movement to involve and empower consumers also adds a new dimension of complexity to these organizations as they struggle to reconfigure the lines of communication and authority among all stakeholders.

Programmatic Development

In addition to the broad political, economic, technological, social, and cultural forces that are impinging on mental health and human services, there are also specific programmatic developments that are shaping the experience of human services consumers and workers. Chief among these influences are the following.

Providing Services in a Least Restrictive Setting   Deinstitutionalization and the movement to establish community-based services have significantly altered how and where services are provided. While there is considerable debate about the quantity and quality of existing community services, there is little doubt that the locus of services has shifted significantly during the past several decades (Carling, 1995; Means and Smith, 1994; Torrey, 1997).

Holistic Services   The philosophy of providing comprehensive, continuous, and coordinated services has been popular for a long time. Only recently have these concepts been put into practice. Mental health and other human services organizations are employing comprehensive assessment and service planning processes staffed by interdisciplinary teams and implemented with the assistance of case managers to serve individuals and families in a more holistic and responsive manner (Stroul, 1996; Tomlinson and Carrier, 1996). This shift to providing comprehensive, integrated services has forced human services practitioners and organizations to significantly alter the manner in which they function. Working collaboratively with families as well as other providers and agencies requires individuals and organizations to utilize sophisticated communication, problem-solving, and teamwork skills.

Individualized and Family-oriented Services   In response to the general consumer movement as well as concerns expressed by human services advocates, providers are increasingly tailoring their service programs to the individual needs of clients and their families. Rather than fitting individuals into prepackaged service programs, some human services agencies are encouraging staff to engage in more flexible and creative service planning. The related development is the emphasis on involving and responding to needs of the whole family rather than the identified client (Adams and Nelson, 1995).

Managed Care   No trend in human services has evoked more controversy in recent years than the introduction of managed care. Initially instituted to curtail the rapidly rising costs of health care, managed care techniques are currently being applied in a variety of human services domains with stated purposes ranging from improving the appropriateness and quality of service to achieving greater efficiency. Critics of early managed care initiatives objected to the negative consequences of limiting benefits and access to service and the single-minded focus on the bottom line at the expense of service quality and consumer choice. Although more recent managed care initiatives place greater emphasis on issues of service and quality, it is difficult to predict how managed care will evolve and what its impact will be on consumers and providers of human services (Kunnes, 1994; Oliver, 1998).

And Other Pressures of Modern Life   The primary message of this chapter is that it is not sufficient for persons entering the fields of mental health and other human services to be equipped only with a desire to help others; a conceptual framework that allows one to understand the causes and remediation of emotional, behavioral, and social problems; and a set of pertinent clinical and programmatic tools. It is also important to understand the context in which one is working. This includes both the particular organization or service delivery system in which one is functioning and the larger environment that impinges on that organizational entity. Tucker (1991) identifies ten important driving forces of change that contemporary businesses must take into account to ensure their survival. While some of these factors have been addressed earlier in this chapter, a brief summary of these driving forces may emphasize the depth and complexity of the change process and its impact on human services consumers, practitioners, and organizations.

• *Speed*   The pace of change—both technological and social—continues to accelerate. Computers appear to become obsolete shortly after they are unpacked. New medications and medical procedures are introduced with great frequency. Even the rate at which pop cultures replace each other seems to be accelerating, as evidenced by the rapid change in musical tastes and clothing styles among young people.

While selected functions within human services are performed at a rapid pace—such as crisis intervention—most practitioners historically have been accustomed to functioning at a more moderate tempo, working methodically over a sustained period of time to facilitate personal growth in clients or restructure dysfunctional environments. Modalities directed at individual change—such as psychotherapy—and system interventions—including neighborhood and community development initiatives—were not expected to produce instant results. Practitioners and, in many instances, consumers understood that it would take considerable time, often years, for these approaches to achieve meaningful change.

Today, with technological advances and the heightened expectations of payors and consumers of services, practitioners are expected to produce tangible results within a brief period of time. Managed care entities emphasize brief treatment modalities and measurable outcomes. Executive and legislative bodies have little patience for explanations of the economic and social complexities of poverty. They are tired of the failed efforts of the past and want recipients of public aid to move quickly from welfare rolls to gainful employment.

Not only have practitioners been forced to adopt new modalities such as brief therapy, but they are also being held accountable for producing tangible results more quickly. The stress of having to work at a more rapid pace and, for many individuals and organizations, to assume greater financial risk has taken a significant toll on many human services practitioners and administrators.

• *Convenience*   In addition to expecting a more rapid response, payors and recipients of assistance also expect services to be delivered in a friendlier, more convenient manner. In response to these trends, human services providers are reassessing traditions that are not especially responsive to consumer and family needs. In order to become more "customer friendly," agencies are attempting to shorten their response time, that is, to reduce long waiting periods for appointments, provide more information about the rationale and purpose of service interventions, and allow consumers and family more involvement in the planning and delivery of services at the individual and program levels. A New Orleans urologist has reoriented his practice to be more responsive to patients by scheduling appointments based on the length of time required for procedures to be given during the visit (Tucker, 1991). This physician has relabeled the waiting room, referring to it as a reception room, and does not charge patients for visits if they are not seen within twenty minutes of their scheduled appointment time.

• *Age Waves*   Each generation has its own set of cultural expectations and preferences. With increased longevity and a more rapid pace of change, service providers are confronted with a greater array of needs and lifestyles.

Increased mobility and reduction in the size of the average family have diminished the role of the extended family for persons at all stages of life. Grandparents are less available to serve as caretakers for their children's off-spring. Conversely, fewer families are inclined to care for elderly members in their homes. This has created greater demand for human services organizations to serve as surrogate caretakers who can fill these gaps.

Each generation has unique needs and assets. The mature market is not only the most rapidly growing sector of the population but also controls the lion's share of the nation's financial resources, with persons over age fifty-five having four times greater median net worth than individuals less than age fifty-five (U.S. Bureau of the Census, 1993). Human services organizations are increasingly orienting services to older individuals due to the size and wealth of this population. At the other end of the chronological continuum are young people growing up in an environment of rapid change, a widening rift between the "haves and have nots," and a high prevalence of substance abuse and violence. The stress experienced by these youngsters poses a formidable challenge to human services agencies.

• *Lifestyle*   Changes in lifestyle have relevance for human services organizations both as indicators of consumer desire and need, and as characteristics of the current and future workforce. As individuals become more reliant on computers and other modern forms of information processing, consumers of services are turning to this technology to gain information and knowledge, for example, on the Internet. With the enhanced capability of interactive communication, consumers are likely to use this technology as a vehicle for receiving services as well as a reference and referral source.

The vocational and personal lifestyles of workers are also changing. For example, in a large-scale survey of U.S. workers, respondents were asked to identify the reasons they considered to be very important in taking their current job. The three most frequently cited factors were (1) open communication, (2) the effect on family and personal life, and (3) the nature of the work, while salary and advancement opportunities ranked fifteenth and sixteenth in frequency of response (Shellenbarger, 1993).

• *Choice*   As consumers become more sophisticated, they expect to have greater input regarding where and how they receive services. This became evident in the heated dialogues that have occurred on the subject of managed health care. While much of the concern expressed by consumers and professionals was focused on the issue of reduced availability of resources, strong opposition has also been voiced whenever managed care entities have proposed curtailing the ability of service recipients to choose their health-care providers or the range of services available to them. While the movement to contain costs remains strong, noticeable shifts in allowing consumers a greater degree of latitude in choosing service providers have occurred.

• *Discounting*   Until recently, human services professionals typically did not devote much attention to fiscal matters. Therapists generally did not speak to patients about paying their bills, and direct services staff did not worry about the sources and amounts of revenue their agencies received. Human services workers assumed that if they had provided good services, they did not have to worry about the stability of their programs or the security of their jobs. All of this has changed as government officials and other funding sources have become concerned about the rising costs of services and as financial support has become more difficult to obtain. Providers that have been accustomed to charging for the actual cost of their services, plus some margin for growth or profit, are now finding themselves in the position of having to reduce fees in order to remain competitive. Agencies have been forced to eliminate positions or reduce salaries, and practitioners have become more conscious about the connection between services and funding.

• *Adding Value and Customer Service*   Cost is not the only factor that enters into a consumer's or payor's decision about where to obtain services. The context in which service is provided is also important. Taking a trip to your local supermarket may help you to understand this point. If you ask an employee where to find an item, you are likely to receive one of three responses. The employee will (1) shrug and tell you that he or she doesn't know, (2) tell you the aisle number and point you in the right direction, or (3) walk with you to where the item is or to someone who can take you to the correct location. Your perception of the store and your inclination to continue to shop there again may be significantly influenced by how the employee responds to your request. There is a high degree of probability that the response you receive is not accidental or simply a reflection of the employee's personality. Managers of successful stores understand the importance of treating customers in a friendly and helpful manner. They devote considerable effort to ensuring that employees make this principle operational in their everyday behavior.

The attitude of service providers toward consumers, the manner in which consumers are treated, and other less tangible aspects of service delivery become more critical to a service organization's success as consumer expectations rise and competition increases. In contrast to supermarkets, human services providers are unlikely to provide discount coupons and free samples. However, there are other methods for adding value and enhancing customer service within the human services that increase customer satisfaction and also may contribute directly to positive outcomes. For example, families have historically been excluded and even rejected by child-caring agencies such as child welfare and mental health, based on the belief that families were to blame for their children's problems (Cohen, Singh, Hosick, and Tremaine, 1992). Many agencies are redefining the role of the family within their service system and are attempting to develop "family-friendly" service approaches, treating families as partners rather than as adversaries.

• *Technical Edge*   Earlier in this chapter we discussed the influence of technology on human services and society. Examples of how technology can aid service providers in improving effectiveness and efficiency include the following:

Use of appointment-scheduling computer programs to enhance access to services

Introduction of electronic recordkeeping to reduce reliance on paper

Availability of interactive telecommunications to bring expertise to sparsely populated regions

• *Quality:*   In mental health and other human services, quality is often mentioned and rarely measured. Admittedly it is difficult to codify quality in these fields; it is not, however, impossible. One promising approach is to use outcome measures as indicators of quality. Lyons et al. (1997) identify several factors that have contributed to the increased emphasis on outcome management in mental health:

Managed care organizations   In its early stages of development, managed care was almost exclusively concerned with reducing costs. More recently, in response to complaints from consumers and other stakeholders, managed care entities have focused attention on managing the quality of care received by clients. They have used outcome measures such as client functioning, symptom reduction, and consumer satisfaction to assess the effectiveness of services.

Consumer movement   As consumer advocacy organizations have grown in strength, their concerns about issues of quality and value have received more attention at national and local levels.

Information technology   Advances in computer capacity have enabled providers and evaluators to process service evaluation data and findings more rapidly. As access to evaluation information is made easier, administrators and practitioners are better able to incorporate this feedback into service planning and modification efforts.

The changing business culture   As business organizations, including health-care entities, shift toward internally driven strategies for self-improvement, the historical reliance on external evaluations is diminishing (Hersey, Blanchard, and Johnson, 1996). Behavioral health-care organizations are now making greater use of clinical outcome and utilization data to help them improve performance and remain viable in a constantly changing market (Lyons et al., 1997).

PERSPECTIVE AND BALANCE
EASY TO DESCRIBE, HARDER TO ACHIEVE

How can we cope with the multiple forces of change described above? What can we do to achieve a reasonable balance between dealing with the demands of personal and family life and the multiple stresses experienced at work? Within human services, are we at risk of losing our focus on helping individuals and families as we become immersed in the political and economic issues that pervade human services?

As the pace and scope of change increase, we are not only being asked to move more quickly, but we are often being pushed in more than one direction at the same time. How do we reconcile competing goals and establish priorities that allow us to be productive and compassionate while maintaining our own mental health?

Reconciling the multiple demands that confront us is no easy task. When the forces that impact human services conflict with each other, it becomes even more difficult to remain on a rational and consistent course. Consider the following: Advances in communication technology and the increased permeability of organizational boundaries have made us more interdependent on each other. At the same time, our reliance on technology and the increased emphasis on achieving bottom-line targets tend to make us more self-absorbed and isolated. In the same vein, the pressure to be more productive will at some point interfere with another current priority: the active involvement of workers in determining how to best provide services. Finding the time and energy to be creative while confronted with increased demand for greater efficiency requires enormous stamina and skill.

If we are to be successful in today's complex environment, it is important to understand the forces that shape human services policy and practice. Understanding that cost-containment and accountability initiatives are driven by an historical absence of documented support for the effectiveness and efficiency of service programs is important. Knowing how to use that information constructively within the work setting is a different matter. In recent years many authors have offered advice on how to cope with complex and stressful work situations (Covey, 1990; Peters, 1994). Most of the reputable experts discourage people from following a simple prescription or formula. Instead they recommend that each person develop a conceptual framework and set of practical strategies that allows one to maintain a rational perspective regarding what is within one's control and what is not while taking care of one's own physical, emotional, and spiritual well-being and learning to accept the inevitability of continual change.

POINTS TO PONDER

1. If human services theory and practice are directly influenced by prevailing political and economic forces, what do you consider to be the emerging political and economic trends in our society? How do you think these will be reflected in human services practice within the next few years?

2. The current emphasis on customer satisfaction is certainly consistent with the fundamental goals of human services. What strategies can be used to enhance the responsiveness of human services organizations to their clientele? What are some of the obstacles that need to be overcome to achieve this goal?

3. As enhanced technology and contemporary management philosophy propel us toward a global economy, communication and interaction patterns have changed dramatically. How are these changes affecting human services organizations? What implications does this have regarding how we prepare personnel to work in this field?

4. The current focus on diversity in our society has serious implications for the field of human services. How can practitioners and service organizations better accommodate the unique interests, needs, and strengths of the multiple racial, ethnic, gender, and sexual orientation groups that seek services? What consideration should be given to staff selection and training, as well as the design and provision of services?

CLASSROOM TO COMMUNITY

Applying the Concepts of Change

- Select a human services organization with which you are familiar. Identify the political, economic, social, and technological forces that are impacting the structure and function of this organization. Describe how these forces have affected the services, clients, staff, and operation of the organization.

CHAPTER 2

APPLYING ORGANIZATIONAL DEVELOPMENT AND LEADERSHIP THEORIES

Our idea of power is changing. Men have long worshiped power; the power of arms, the power of divine right—of kings or priests—and then in the nineteenth century the power of majorities. Our conception of democracy is only today beginning to free itself from that taint. . . . Power is now beginning to be thought of by some as the combined capacities of a group. We get power through effective relations. This means that some people are beginning to conceive of the leader, not as the man in the group who is able to assert his individual will and get others to follow him, but as the one who knows how to relate these different wills so that they will have a driving force. He must know how to create group power rather than to express a personal power. He must make the team.

⁓ Mary Parker Follett, *Dynamic Administration: The Collected Papers of Mary Parker Follett* , 1948

Increased demands for flexibility, accountability, and productivity have forced human services providers to reexamine the manner in which they deliver services. Adapting to the evolving human services environment requires not only greater operational efficiency but also fundamental changes in values and orientation. In order to be responsive to fiscal constraints, technological innovation, and consumer needs, human services organizations are turning to the experience and literature of the business sector, which has undergone radical transformation during the past two decades.

In this chapter we describe recent trends in developing and managing organizations. We discuss similarities and differences between business and human services organizations and raise questions about how human services organizations can maintain their focus on responding to the needs of people while remaining fiscally viable. We examine organizational behavior and its relationship to human services and describe some of the conceptual approaches that have been used to explain and modify organizational behavior. We also explore strategies for enabling organizations to function effectively in a complex and rapidly changing environment. In addition, we address some of the critical issues that human services organizations are currently confronting and discuss how organizations can best deal with these issues in order to ensure the provision of effective services while supporting the workers responsible for providing these services.

~

COMPLEX ORGANIZATIONS IN A COMPLEX SOCIETY

In today's complex society, human services are rarely provided by a single individual. Even a solo practitioner is dependent on other individuals and organizations. A physician in private practice needs someone to schedule appointments, handle patient billing, and keep the examination rooms clean and safe. This physician is also likely to employ a nurse to assist in conducting many of the diagnostic treatment procedures. Also, unless his or her clientele are extremely wealthy, the physician will be dependent on insurance companies, managed care entities, and other third-party payors for financial support.

The provision of even the most basic human services has become a complex ordeal involving not only the consumer and provider but also an array of entities engaged in supporting, financing, and regulating these services. Each of these functions is typically carried out within an organizational context, and each organization must interact with the others on a regular basis. It follows that how well services are provided is dependent to a large extent on how each organization functions and how the various entities relate to each other.

Early theories of management and organizational behavior placed managers in a strict hierarchical relationship to workers. The job of the manager was to supervise and motivate workers as well as to organize tasks to increase efficiency and productivity (Fayol, 1949; Gantt, 1974; Taylor, 1911). As our society shifted from being centered around family and village to a broader urban culture based on technology, the way in which we viewed organizations also changed.

We are no longer enamored by linear solutions to organizational challenges. Top-down management control may provide clear direction, but it does not take into account the importance of motivational factors that influence workers' performance. Technology is an important resource but cannot by itself ensure an organization's success. Managers need to be sensitive to the multiple internal and external forces that impact an organization's performance. Hersey et al. (1996) describe three variables that determine organizational effectiveness:

1. *Causal variables.*   These factors are within the organization's control and include leadership strategies, skills and behavior, management decisions, and the policy and structure of the organization.

2. *Intervening variables.*   These factors include the current condition of the internal state of the organization, such as the commitment to objectives, motivation, and morality of its members and their skills in communication and conflict resolution.

3. *Output or end results variables.*   These variables reflect the achievement of the organization and include quantity and quality of services produced.

Hersey et al. note that most managers look solely at output measures such as profit, win-loss records, and number of goods or services produced. If causal or intervening factors are overlooked, long-term performance will inevitably suffer. Contemporary organizations have to deal not only with factors within their own work settings but also need to attend to the variety of political, economic, and social forces emanating from their external environments.

MANAGING CONTEMPORARY ORGANIZATIONS

Organizations may be viewed as social systems composed of many interrelated subsystems. The changes in one system affect changes in other parts of the total system. Following are the primary organizational subsystems (Hersey et al., 1996):

1. human social
2. administrative/structural
3. information/decision making
4. economic/technological

Today we recognize not only the complexity of organizations but also their fluidity. A stable organization may suddenly be thrown into a state of crisis as a result of an economic downswing or change in public policy. A management style that works in one situation may not work in another (Blake and Mouton, 1994). This recognition has led to the development of leadership and management approaches that take into account personal and situational differences. One approach that acknowledges variation in management style as well as the differential impact of each style is the managerial grid developed

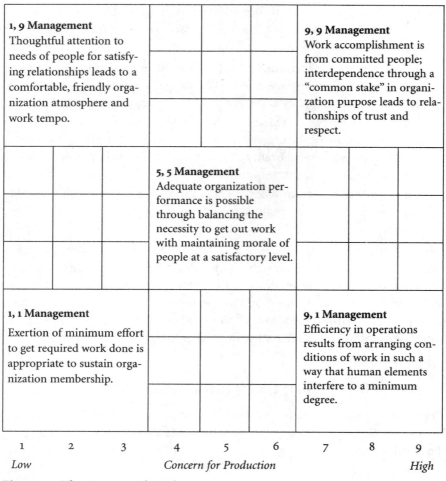

1, 9 Management
Thoughtful attention to needs of people for satisfying relationships leads to a comfortable, friendly organization atmosphere and work tempo.

9, 9 Management
Work accomplishment is from committed people; interdependence through a "common stake" in organization purpose leads to relationships of trust and respect.

5, 5 Management
Adequate organization performance is possible through balancing the necessity to get out work with maintaining morale of people at a satisfactory level.

1, 1 Management
Exertion of minimum effort to get required work done is appropriate to sustain organization membership.

9, 1 Management
Efficiency in operations results from arranging conditions of work in such a way that human elements interfere to a minimum degree.

| 1 | 2 | 3 | 4 | 5 | 6 | 7 | 8 | 9 |

Low   *Concern for Production*   *High*

Figure 1   The Managerial Grid

by Blake and Mouton (1994). This grid, depicted in Figure 1, describes managerial styles based on an individual's concern for people or production. Blake and Mouton explain how individuals at different places on this continuum might handle creativity and change in organizations. For example, a manager whose style places a high value on production with little concern for persons may respond quickly to innovations. At the subordinate level, however, if there is little opportunity for creativity, employees either become disinterested or all of their creative thinking goes into undermining the system and preventing it from working well. Conversely, under a manager who is primarily focused on people with little concern for productivity, the boss is likely to have low aspirations for creativity and, at the subordinate level, individuals are likely to be highly committed to their superiors. This commitment, however, is in the human direction. Because productivity is not highly valued, there is no built-in motivation for creativity, and change is only likely to be accepted if others support it.

In a scenario where concern for both productivity and people is low, the boss may be creative in other domains of life—but not at work—and will probably dampen the efforts to be creative of those at the subordinate level. Some subordinates may prefer this managerial style to a low-production/high-personal concern or a moderate-production/moderate-personal concern orientation. The low-personal/low-production concern orientation encourages delegation, allowing the individual to freely pursue work activities to achieve his or her commitments.

When concern for both person and production are high, the manager is typically an experimenter and innovator. The manager stimulates subordinates and pays close attention to good ideas regardless of who expresses them. Because the aim is to improve how work is done rather than change for change sake, and participation and involvement in work activities are encouraged, innovation in this organizational setting is more likely to arise.

Blake and Mouton assert that an individual's management style may vary from one situation to another. The style that is dominant for a particular person in a given situation is influenced by one or several sets of the following conditions:

- Organizational practices that encourage or inhibit a particular managerial style.
- The situational context that exists at the moment. Management of people will be different in crisis and routine circumstances.
- The values of the individual, especially those related to the proper way to treat people or achieve results.
- The deeply rooted personality characteristics that might incline an individual to improve a particular style.
- Chance. A person who has not been exposed to a particular style may be less likely to adopt that managerial orientation than someone who has awareness of a variety of managerial styles.

APPLYING SYSTEMS AND MANAGEMENT PRINCIPLES

Providing effective human services in the current environment is a formidable challenge. Included among the factors that make this a difficult endeavor are the magnitude of human needs and problems, the complexity of modern society and its institutions, and the current reluctance of the public to devote additional resources to human services. Operating in a context of rapid change adds another degree of complexity to the service delivery process. A number of systems approaches have been developed in the latter part of the twentieth century in order to aid managers and organizations to respond to this complex set of dynamics. The aim of these system approaches is to bring the need of the organization and the need of the individual closer together (Huse, 1980).

Many of the management approaches that have emerged in the United States during the last decade have been responses to the extraordinary success of Japanese businesses. It is interesting to note that some of the techniques used by Japanese businesses were attempted and rejected by the United States in the 1950s (Bowditch and Buono, 1985). These techniques were introduced to the Japanese by W. Edwards Demming (1982, 1986) and his colleagues and then refined by Kaoru Ishikawa (1985). One of the central concepts of this plan was the quality control circle, which was introduced as a program to improve the quality of services through the input of employees. A quality circle is a small group of workers who meet regularly to discuss ways to improve quality. These workers are paid overtime for meetings after work with a supervisor. This process encourages employee participation in the organization and the exchange of ideas.

Total quality management (TQM) is a systems approach that promotes employee participation as a vehicle to implement companywide principles and practices to ensure complete customer satisfaction. Each individual in the organization is seen as both a customer and a supplier of goods, services, or information and may play both roles in the same transaction (Moss, 1996). For example, a caseworker who serves welfare clients relies on the business office of the department of social services to provide the clients' food stamps and subsidy checks. The caseworker is a supplier to the client and a customer of the business office. This perspective focuses on the relationship between different elements of an organization as well as the relationship between the organization and its consumers. Another key factor of TQM is the requirement of continuous improvement. Theorists recognize that restructuring takes time and will not last if a one-shot attempt is made. Every member of the organization is charged with the responsibilities of self-reflection and consideration of the larger picture. All members examine the causes of problems and work to develop solutions.

An outgrowth of total quality management is organization engineering (Hammer and Champy, 1993; Champy, 1995). While total quality management focuses on incremental improvement through creative interaction among employees, reengineering focuses on overhauling the manner in which a corporation operates. A mental health organization employing a TQM approach might attempt to reduce the waiting period between a patient applying for services and actually being seen. Proponents of reengineering would be more inclined to restructure the entire service delivery process to achieve desired outcomes. While TQM and reengineering share common characteristics such as employee participation, customer satisfaction, increased efficiency, and redistribution of power, reengineering is a more ambitious and revolutionary approach. The shift from TQM to reengineering mirrors the general societal trend of expecting larger and quicker results.

Corporate organizational theory is more relevant to human services than ever before. As the climate changes, organizations must learn to operate in the most efficient and cost-effective ways. Many of the concerns of businesses as they undergo reengineering and restructuring are now recognized as critical issues for human services organizations (Adams and Nelson, 1995; Drucker, 1990; Osborne and Gaebler, 1992; Osborne and Plastrik, 1997).

With recent dramatic reductions in funding support, community-based not-for-profit organizations are operating in an immensely different and far more challenging environment than previously encountered. Such organizations now face critical issues of survival and drastic downsizing with minimal resources and significant restraints. Many are having to make tough choices—to close or reorganize programs, to reduce staff, to sell facilities or terminate leases. Others are working to ensure the future of their programs by merging with other groups or advocating for change in regulations and legislation.

The traditional distinctions between human services and business are fading. The large amount of money—both public and private—that is expended on human services has caused consumers, financial institutions, and government to demand greater accountability from service providers. As the private sector moves into domains that were traditionally the exclusive domain of not-for-profit organizations—corrections and public education, for example—greater emphasis is placed on productivity and competition. Government and other not-for-profit service providers are finding that they have to become more businesslike if they wish to survive.

With adoption of corporate strategies and approaches has arisen an understandable expression of concern that human services organizations, in their eagerness to attend to the well-being of the bottom line, may sacrifice their core values of compassion and commitment to caring for persons regardless of their economic status. As with all other aspects of contemporary organizational functioning, maintaining a balance between providing person- and family-centered services while adopting good management practices takes considerable skill and fortitude. Achieving this balance requires intelligent and strong leadership.

Although many of the approaches that are being applied in human services were first used in business settings, it would be inaccurate to conclude that the influence is unidirectional. Many of the basic concepts employed in organizational development are borrowed from psychology and social science, and the emphasis on interpersonal relationships has long been a hallmark of human services.

THE NEW LEADER

As we learn more about effective management, the definition of a good leader is evolving. No longer is the monolithic model considered ideal. Rather, people skills are as important as business knowledge in today's market. One of the most significant trends in management is the idea of the leader as inspirational, as an innovator. That leader does not exist simply to rule in a hierarchy but rather to guide his or her workers.

Considerable attention has been given to the importance of having visionary leaders (Bennis, 1989; Peters and Waterman, 1982). These are individuals who see beyond the constraints of the status quo and are able to communicate to all members of the organization not only the importance and value of their vision but also the plausibility of actualizing this vision if everyone works together. Leaders are viewed as having attributes distinctly different from traditional managers (see Table 1).

Recently, organizational theorists and practitioners have focused attention on levels of management below the chief executive officer, president, or director of an organization. Recognizing that genuine change requires more than vision and inspiration, these individuals have focused on transforming managers from implementers to change agents. Katzenbach et al. (1995) list seven attributes of real change leaders, individuals who are able to create growth and high performance in organizational settings:

- Commitment to a better way
- Courage to challenge existing power bases and norms
- Personal initiative to go beyond defined boundaries
- Motivation of themselves and others

TABLE 1   Differences Between Managers and Leaders

The Manager:	**The Leader:**
Administers	Innovates
Is a copy	Is an original
Maintains	Develops
Focuses on systems and structure	Focuses on people
Relies on control	Inspires trust
Has a short-range view	Has a long-range perspective
Asks how and when	Asks what and why
Has eye always on the bottom line	Has eye on the horizon
Imitates	Originates
Accepts the status quo	Challenges it
Is the classic good soldier	Is own person
Does things right	Does the right thing

W. Bennis, *On Becoming a Leader* (p. 45) copyright © 1989 by Warren Bennis, Inc. Reprinted by permission of Addison Wesley Longman.

- Caring about how people are treated and enabled to perform
- Staying undercover—keeping attention on the process and goal rather than the individual manager
- A sense of humor about themselves and their situation

Effective organizational leaders—in both human services and corporate cultures—recognize that their most valuable resources are the individuals who work in their organizations. Even organizations dependent on sophisticated technology will not perform well if staff are not properly trained and sufficiently motivated. Contemporary organizational approaches acknowledge the importance of respecting and involving workers. They also demand a great deal from staff. Business as usual does not exist in the realm of total quality management or reengineering. Moving from a product orientation to a people-oriented philosophy requires that workers not only exercise physical and technical skills but also become active participants in improving work processes and responding to the needs of consumers. Contemporary leaders and managers play a critical role in engaging workers and empowering staff to become active stakeholders in the process, contributing through their problem-solving, customer relations, and change-agent efforts as well as being productive workers.

SELECTING THE RIGHT TOOL FOR THE JOB

Commenting on a hospital director who had successfully reformed a large state psychiatric facility in his first assignment, but was unable to function effectively in his second post as a chief executive officer, Levine and Perkins (1997) observed, "The lesson is that methods must be adopted to the historical situation and to conditions as they exist." Recognizing that one size does not fit all, Hersey and Blanchard developed a model of situational leadership in the late 1960s (Hersey and Blanchard, 1969). The basic premise of this model is that there is not a single best way to influence people. The nature of the work to be performed, the demands of the environment—internal and external, and the level of preparation of followers are the critical variables that should be considered in selecting an appropriate leadership style. To assist individuals in organizations to determine the most effective style of leadership for particular situations, situational leadership offers a framework based on the interrelationship among the following (Hersey et al., 1996):

1. The degree of guidance and direction provided by a leader (task behavior)
2. The amount of socioemotional support a leader gives (relationship behavior)
3. The readiness level followers demonstrate in carrying out a specific task, function, or objective

Readiness has two major components: ability and willingness. In this context, willingness refers to level of confidence, commitment, and motivation to accomplish a particular task.

A central tenet of the situational leadership model is the importance of the follower in determining whether leadership will be effective. Hersey et al. also observe that leaders do not possess power without it being given to them by their followers.

The situational leadership model might be applied in human services settings characterized by varying levels of readiness. Hersey et al. describe four leadership styles.

- Style 1 (S1). This leadership style is characterized by above-average amounts of task behavior and below-average amounts of relationship behavior.
- Style 2 (S2). This leadership style is characterized by above-average amounts of both task behavior and relationship behavior.
- Style 3 (S3). This style is characterized by above-average amounts of relationship behavior and below-average amounts of task behavior.

- Style 4 (S4). This style is characterized by below-average amounts of both relationship behavior and task behavior.

In a crisis situation it may be most appropriate to respond with an S1 leadership approach. For instance, if a group of children in a day treatment program begins to fight with each other, it is more important for the supervisor to make sure that staff intervene quickly and appropriately. Providing staff with encouragement and support at that moment would probably not help to stabilize the situation. Once the crisis has passed, it would be appropriate to provide emotional support and encourage workers to reassess intervention strategy. Similarly, the leader of an organization faced with an imminent reduction of funding needs to take steps to deal with the threat to the organization and may not have the time to solicit the feelings and opinions of staff.

While S1 is typically referred to as a telling approach because the leader provides specific instructions and supervises performance closely, S2 is sometimes referred to as a selling approach. In the scenario of the organization threatened by funding reduction, the leader might use an S2 approach once the decisions have been made regarding how the organization will respond to this threat. By explaining the decisions that have been made and offering opportunities for clarification, the leader elicits buy-in from the employees. The S2 leadership style would be appropriate in a situation where individuals or groups are confident and willing to try to accomplish tasks but are not yet able to do so, such as a group of teachers learning a new social studies curriculum who might benefit from intensive instruction accompanied by considerable emotional support and encouragement.

The S3 style of leadership is appropriate when the individual or group is unable to perform but may be willing or confident. In situations where the follower has recently developed an ability and has not had the chance yet to gain confidence by taking action on his or her own or is able and willing but has low motivation, the leader might not provide much guidance but would engage in high amounts of two-way communication and supportive behavior. This leadership style might be appropriate in a social welfare agency in which staff are angry at their supervisor because of policy changes that have been instituted which they believe are unreasonable. They are capable of performing their work but are resisting the changes taking place. In this situation, the supervisor would want to facilitate a process that would address the employees' concerns while ensuring that the work of the agency is accomplished. This style of leadership, which is referred to as participating, involves considerable supporting and empowering on the part of the leader.

The S4 style of leadership, which in many ways represents the highest level of development, is characterized by low guidance and low supportive behavior. The use of this style, which is referred to as a delegating approach, is appropriate when followers are both able and willing to perform their work. The leader feels comfortable turning over responsibility for decisions and implementation to followers. William Bratton, Police Commissioner of New York City from 1994 to 1996, employed this leadership style to decentralize decision making and control to a local level. He asserts that the dramatic improvement in public safety in New York City witnessed in the mid 1990s was due, in large part, to his willingness to delegate authority to the precinct and individual officer level (Bratton with Knobler, 1998). When followers are genuinely able and willing to assume responsibility, the leader can best serve by allowing them to be self-directed. In this style, leadership performs by observing and monitoring the followers' performance. If followers are not ready, however, this form of leadership is likely to result in poor performance and organizational dysfunction.

These four leadership styles are not designed to be applied in a formulaic manner. Their value lies in reminding us that the best leadership approaches are those that are compatible with the needs and demands of a particular situation. In the situational leadership model, consistency is not defined as using the same style all the time. Instead, consistency refers to using the same style in all similar situations but adapting the style appropriately in response to situational changes (Hersey et al., 1996).

COPING SUCCESSFULLY WITH CHANGE

Much has been written about the characteristics of successful leaders and corporations (Drucker, 1992, 1993, 1995; Peters, 1985). Most of this material stresses the importance of having a clear vision of what the organization wants (and does not want) to be, developing a strategic plan of how to actualize this vision, and being prepared to work hard to implement the plan. Other attributes that are frequently mentioned are positive, effective, and continuous communication, the ability to be flexible, and creativity. Finally, most experts emphasize the importance of taking care of oneself, recognizing the signs of burnout, attending to one's physical, mental, emotional, and spiritual well-being, and allowing adequate time for self-renewal.

One of the most articulate proponents of self-development is Steven Covey who has written extensively about the seven habits of highly effective people (Covey, 1990). Covey believes that effective people have acquired patterns of behavior involving three overlapping components: knowledge, attitude, and skills. He believes that the habits of behavior that enable these individuals to be effective are learned and not innate, and he suggests that individuals focus on developing the following habits:

1. *Be proactive.* Effective people take responsibility for their attitudes and actions. By exercising the freedom to choose responses based on their values and decisions rather than on their moods and conditions, they become proactive.

2. *Begin with an end in mind.* Effective people have a clear understanding of where they want to be, not only in the long run but also on a daily basis. They use their specific purpose as a basis for making decisions and are clear on their values and priorities prior to selecting goals and conducting their business.

3. *Put first things first.* Effective people decide what is important and act on these priorities. Importance is not defined simply by urgency but also by other personal priorities that we deem to be personally valuable.

4. *Think win-win.* Effective people seek mutual benefit. Success is best achieved when people work collaboratively.

5. *Seek first to understand, then to be understood.* Effective people are empathic and seek to understand the point of view of the other person before expressing their own interests and desires.

6. *Synergize.* Effective people actively engage in creative cooperation and teamwork. Bringing a variety of perspectives together in an atmosphere of mutual respect allows one to explore a greater range of possibilities and to ultimately select the best approach.

7. *Sharpen the saw.* Effective people systematically pursue a balanced program of self-renewal directed at the body, mind, emotions, and spirit.

CHANGE AS LOSS

One of the significant contributions of human services practice theory to the study of organizational change is its explanation of how individuals cope with the stress of change. Borrowing from Kubler-Ross's (1981) psychological theory of the stages of grief, organizational development specialists have postulated that change is equivalent to loss for individuals who are confronted with significant modification of their work situations. These individuals may not only resist such changes, but they will go through a process similar to mourning in the course of adjusting to change. The initial reaction of denial will be followed by anger and depression prior to the person's acceptance of the change. Sadly, some individuals are so devastated by change that they cannot accept what has occurred. These individuals may experience serious emotional distress that prevents them from adapting to change and moving on with their lives.

Fortunately, the distress associated with change is usually transitional. However, the pain experienced is real, and an individual's inability to adjust may significantly disrupt an organization's performance. Effective leaders are sensitive to the impact of change on workers and customers and will build into the change process mechanisms for assisting individuals to work through these changes. Providing information on why change is occurring and how it will proceed is useful. Offering opportunities for individuals to express their feelings about the changes and to receive support during the course of change may also be beneficial. Enlightened organizations will give stakeholders the opportunity for input about the changes that are being considered, especially in the areas that directly impact them.

Major change is never without difficulty or consequence. However, those responsible for implementing change can buffer some of its effect by engaging individuals in the process and offering them opportunity to shape the future of the organization.

CREATING EFFECTIVE HUMAN SERVICES PROGRAMS

There have also been attempts to describe effective programs in the field of human services. Schorr has identified seven attributes of highly effective programs (1997).

1. Successful programs are comprehensive, flexible, responsive, and persevering.
2. Successful programs see children in the context of their families.
3. Successful programs deal with families as parts of neighborhood and communities.
4. Successful programs have a long-term preventive orientation and a clear mission, and they continue to evolve over time.
5. Successful programs are well-managed by competent and committed individuals with clearly identifiable skills.
6. Staff of successful programs are trained and supported to provide high-quality, responsive services.
7. Successful programs build strong relationships based on mutual trust and respect.

Addressing the question of why there are not more effective programs, Schorr states that programs are often undermined by their system surroundings. She observes that although there is a growing consensus about what elements make a successful program, there has not been sufficient attention to the issue of how to incorporate the attributes of effectiveness into those institutions and systems into which the program must fit if they are to serve large numbers of people. Small model programs that have demonstrated effectiveness with a few hundred persons are forced to sacrifice many of the critical elements of success when they are adapted to rigid, bureaucratic systems.

MORE THAN BUSINESS AS USUAL

It should be apparent by now that human services organizations share many of the same issues and challenges as their counterparts from the business community. There are, however, distinct differences that begin with the stated missions of the two types of organizations. Although human services organizations have by necessity become more sensitive to the economic realities of their enterprise, the primary mission, for most helping organizations, is to provide services to individuals and families in need of assistance. Many business entities consider service to be a priority. For these organizations, however, the service mission is typically viewed as subordinate to the goal of creating a profit for the company's owners and investors.

The output, or product, of human services organizations is often less tangible than that of a business organization. It is easier to assess the outcome of an automobile manufacturer or a restaurant than it is to judge the quality of a psychotherapeutic intervention. Because the automobile or cheeseburger is usually purchased and paid for directly by the consumer, the business transaction is typically less complicated than one that occurs in the field of human services. One example of this difference is that the financial, social, and technical support provided to welfare recipients is generally paid for by government funds that come from tax revenues. The difficulty associated with measuring how successful these services are and the lack of consensus about the desirability of using public funds to support welfare recipients makes the work of human services administrators and practitioners more difficult.

Hargrove and Glidewell (1990) conducted an interesting analysis of the factors that make human services work in the public sector so difficult. Addressing the challenges faced by executives in public agencies, they provide a conceptual framework for assessing the degree of "impossibility" of various public management jobs. They describe four critical dimensions of difficulty on which the work of public service agencies may be judged. They focus specifically on the role of the agency's chief executive officer, whom they refer to as the commissioner. Their analysis, however, has relevance for everyone involved in that agency's work.

1. *Legitimacy of the Commissioner's Clientele*   The client's degree of legitimacy is determined by two factors: (a) the extent to which people served by the agency are perceived by the public to be responsible, prosocial, and diligent and (b) the extent to which clients are tractable and responsive to the agency's services. Commissioners who serve a responsible clientele such as veterans or farmers, or cooperative, motivated individuals who obviously derive benefits from the services, are more likely to receive public support and will be able to implement plans for change. At the other end of the spectrum, commissioners who serve clientele who are not perceived to be part of mainstream society, or are viewed as unmotivated or unlikely to change, such as criminals and psychiatric patients, will experience considerable difficulty in achieving their goals. When an agency's clientele are seen by the public as irresponsible and intractable, the obstacles to effectively serving this population may be insurmountable.

2. *Intensity of Conflict Among Constituencies*   All human services commissioners or leaders interact with multiple constituencies, including political masters, agency bureaucracy, advocates and opponents of client groups, and the client or regulated group that is the focus of the agency's mission. When conflict among these constituencies is minimal, the job is relatively easy. When groups are in conflict with each other or the commissioner, it becomes much more difficult to achieve desired outcomes. The degree of conflict among constituencies interacts with the legitimacy of the client. For example, all other things being equal, the probability of introducing a new program into the public school environment when there is a mild conflict among the parents, teachers' union, and superintendent of schools is considerably greater than it would be if one were trying to initiate an adult literacy program for welfare recipients with an equivalent degree of conflict among interested constituencies. As Hargrove and Glidewell point out, all conflicts among constituencies are not equal. When the conflict involves moralistic, ideological, or values issues, the conflict is more intense and the leader is likely to elicit a strong negative reaction regardless of whether he or she takes action.

3. *Respect for Professional Authority*   The commissioner's credentials influence the degree of difficulty of that person's job. Leaders of agencies associated with scientifically based professions, such as medicine, are more likely to enjoy the public's respect for their authority and are, therefore, in a better position to overcome public concerns about the legitimacy of clients. A

physician commissioner in a health department, for example, has a less difficult job than the director of a corrections agency who has a degree in public
administration.

4. *Strength of the Agency Myth* When the agency's mission and goals are
widely accepted by the public and have remained stable over a long period of
time, the agency may be said to have a strong myth. A myth may be strong
even if the agency is unlikely to achieve its stated goals. If the agency's missions and goals are unstable and controversial, the myth is weak. An example
of a strong myth is public education. Although constituencies do not expect
complete attainment of educational goals, there is broad acceptance that
almost all children will benefit from education. Because of the strength of
this myth, public education is virtually universal and compulsory. Mental
health, on the other hand, has a relatively weak myth. Treatment philosophies
have shifted periodically regarding whether people should be treated in institutions or in the community, about the efficacy of most treatment modalities, and about just how confusing the field of mental health is to the public,
including executive and legislative leaders.

This particular dimension of difficulty may be used to differentiate public
leadership challenges that have a reasonable chance of being successfully
achieved from those that are unlikely to result in a positive outcome. A commissioner with good professional or scientific credentials who directs an
agency with a well-accepted, enduring myth that serves a legitimate clientele
and has only a few constituencies whose conflicts are relatively minor has a
relatively good chance of succeeding. Examples of public leadership jobs that
are viewed positively ("possible") are public health commissioners and directors of agricultural agencies. At the other end of the spectrum are mental
health, welfare, police, and corrections commissioners whose clientele,
agency myths, and professional authority are viewed negatively by the public
and who deal with multiple constituencies engaged in intense conflict. Individuals who hold these leadership positions are considered to have "impossible" jobs. While these persons may be successful in achieving some of their
agency's goals, implementing significant change requires extraordinary dedication, skill, and support. Even with these assets individuals occupying
impossible public management jobs are likely to have only limited success in
actualizing a vision of reform or even making substantial improvements in
the service delivery system during their tenure.

Hargrove and Glidewell developed this framework in order to sensitize
human services administrators and others to the difficulty of public management jobs and the factors that facilitate or impede a leader's ability to

enhance the performance of human services agencies. This model also provides practical confirmation of the complexity of human services organizations, particularly in relation to their interdependence with the public and multiple constituencies. Successful innovation requires a sophisticated understanding of how these constituencies may react to change and considerable skill in promoting their agenda and reconciling the conflicting positions among the involved parties.

WORKING FROM A POSITION OF STRENGTH

Human services endeavors are generally viewed as problem or deficit oriented. Psychiatrists employ medications to reduce symptoms, while psychotherapists work with individuals and families to modify maladaptive behavioral patterns and eliminate dysfunction. Social workers struggle continuously to control violence, poverty, substance abuse, and a host of other community problems. Educators work with students to overcome learning difficulties, and the police and other justice officials devote considerable energy to controlling and reducing crime.

This problem/deficit orientation is not confined to individual practitioners. As Hargrove and Glidewell (1990) point out, human services agencies are constantly struggling against negative perceptions toward their clients and services. The strong pressures for welfare reform and tougher sentencing of criminals has been driven not only by a belief in the efficacy of these initiatives. The renewed emphasis on punitive approaches is in large part a result of the public's lack of confidence in the agencies charged with serving these individuals and protecting our communities. Human services organizations often find themselves in a reactive posture, defending themselves against attacks from legislative and judicial bodies as well as citizens in the communities in which they are located. This reactive orientation—whether in the context of defending budget appropriations and policy program proposals or combating public stereotypes such as "all persons with mental illness are violent" or "all welfare recipients are lazy"—drains energy and erodes morale. It is little wonder that those who are charged with serving the less fortunate of our society often feel embattled and discouraged. Add to this mix the continual stress of having to adapt to a seemingly endless series of changes, most of which emanate from the external environment, and it is easy to understand why human services practitioners often feel frustrated and discouraged, and their parent organizations appear to be ill prepared to cope with the multiple demands and challenges that confront them.

There is a more promising perspective, one that has the potential of reorganizing human services workers and organizations. In contrast to the problem or deficit perspective, some theorists argue in favor of a strength-based orientation (Apter, 1982; Rutter, 1990; Smale with Tuson, 1992). This positive perspective has found expression both in programs designed to serve clients and models for managing and structuring human services organizations. Some programs such as wraparound care for youth (Yoe et al., 1996) and assertive community treatment for adults with chronic mental illness (Olfson, 1990; Stein and Test, 1980) focus on identifying and supporting the strengths of individual clients as an alternative pathway to coping with disabilities. Kretzmann and McKnight (1993) extend this concept to the community level. They advocate that we can develop strong and healthy communities by mobilizing the assets and capacities of individuals, local associations and organizations, and formal institutions. Rather than viewing people with disabilities and welfare recipients as problem individuals who represent a burden to the community, if we focus on the capacities and abilities of these individuals, they can serve as valuable resources in renewing our beleaguered communities.

At the organizational level, a positive, strength-based orientation is not only more likely to enhance organizational functioning and service delivery—it will also have a positive effect on the attitudes and motivations of individual workers. Sherman (1993), for example, describes strategies for creating the "new American Hospital," which can operate effectively and successfully in today's environment. One of the cornerstones of his strategy for change is the exercise of leadership that recognizes the importance of people as a change element in revitalization. By systematically utilizing recognition, reinforcement, and reward as motivational tools, Sherman believes that hospitals can achieve greater customer satisfaction, quality, productivity, innovation, and profitability.

Sherman does not limit his array of positive strategies to traditional motivational techniques. In addition to advocating for giving pay increases for meritorious performance and encouraging hospitals to promote individuals within their own ranks to higher management positions, he also supports the use of nonfinancial rewards. He suggests that organizations should select the specific behavior that they would like to see exhibited and develop nonfinancial rewards and honors that recognize accomplishments in these areas, such as contributing significantly to a more positive organizational culture. Sending an employee who has exhibited innovative behavior to a training seminar or giving a staff member free tickets to the movies or an athletic event demonstrates the organization's commitment to creativity. He also encourages organizations to have fun, citing laughter and enjoyment as important attributes of a productive and successful organization.

It would be naive to assert that shifting from a deficit to a strength-based perspective will ensure that human services organizations will be able to cope well with change and deliver effective services to their clients. Developing responsive human services organizations is a complex endeavor requiring comprehensive strategic planning, strong leadership, a dedicated workforce, and a community that appreciates the mission and value of the organization. A strength-based perspective does, however, provide important conceptual and practical guidance for any human services organization that wants to sustain its morale and viability while providing support and assistance to its clientele within today's stressful and fluid environment.

POINTS TO PONDER

1. Workers in contemporary organizations are confronted with seemingly competing pressures. The demand for greater productivity places considerable stress on individuals to work quickly and meet continually escalating productivity standards. Contemporary workers are also asked to be more responsive to customers, a task that is obviously more difficult when one is experiencing stress. Describe viable strategies for reducing stress and maintaining focus in a high demand environment. How can organizations help workers to reconcile these potentially diverging priorities?

2. What are the major differences between traditional and contemporary organizational theories? In what ways have these theories been shaped by broader societal factors?

3. Are individuals born good leaders or can leadership be taught or learned? What are the key attributes of a strong leader? What kind of training would facilitate development of individuals to perform leadership roles in today's complex environment?

4. Many contemporary theorists generally agree that one size does not fit all when it comes to organizational communication, management, and leadership. Style varies considerably among individuals, and the same individual may modify his or her approach according to the demands of the situation. What is your preferred style of communication and leadership? In what organizational situations are you most comfortable? What situations cause you the greatest discomfort?

5. With their person-centered focus, it would seem that human services organizations would be well prepared to help workers cope with changes in the internal and external environments. In what ways have human services organizations helped individuals to deal with these changes? How might these organizations improve their performance in this area? Are there lessons that can be learned from the business sector?

6. What are the assets and liabilities of a strength-based approach to human services? How might an organization that currently utilizes a needs- and deficit-based service delivery model modify its approach to incorporate asset- and strength-based strategies? What are the challenges that administration and staff will encounter in making this conversion?

CLASSROOM TO COMMUNITY

Applying the Concepts of Change

- Select a successful organization in your community. What are the characteristics that have enabled the organization to gain this reputation? If possible, ask workers their perceptions of what the organization does to achieve its objectives? Do all individuals share the same views, or are there differences? If there are differences, are these attributable to the workers' positions within the organization?

- Interview individuals in leadership positions in both business and human services organizations. What are the differences and similarities and functions they perform? Are their overall roles in the business and human services sectors more similar or more different? In your opinion, what are the most critical attributes that contributed to the success of these individuals?

DESIGNING CHANGE:
ORGANIZATIONAL PERSPECTIVES

CHAPTER 3

ACTUALIZING THE VISION
Family Services Past and Present

> We have learned from our work that much of the effort
> to help individuals—to which many of us have devoted
> our personal and professional lives—now seems unlikely
> to have a major social effect unless we also face and
> change the forces that make those individuals what they
> are and keep them that way.
>
> ⌒ The Carnegie Council on Children, 1977

A lot of discussion about working with the entire family rather than just attending to the identified client is taking place today. As the following description of the Bridge Program illustrates, this is not a new idea, nor is it a concept that is frequently put into practice. In this chapter, we explore some of the factors that influence an organization's or system's ability to provide family-centered services, and we see how all aspects of the service system influence the nature and quality of the services provided. Having a family-oriented philosophy is important; however, the way in which staff are educated and supported, the funding and incentive mechanisms that are operating, and the political and social forces of the broader community may either impede or contribute to an organization's ability to provide family-centered services. In comparing the success of the Bridge Program, which operated during the 1970s, with current family-oriented initiatives, it becomes apparent that the philosophy and practice of including families in the service plan has been with us for some time and we see how the context in which these services developed has changed significantly during the past several decades. The pace and complexity of the current environment presents challenges to family advocates that did not exist twenty-five years ago.

~

THEN

Winging It

On a sunny afternoon in central New York State in 1970, another young psychologist and I stood outside a rustic lodge and contemplated the future of our new endeavor. We had almost completed conducting staff orientation and training for the Bridge Program Camp, a component of a comprehensive year-round psychoeducational program for children with severe emotional and behavioral problems and their families. The program—established prior to the enactment of Public Law 94–142, which protects the rights of children with special education needs—targeted children between the ages of six and eleven whose troublesome behavior placed them at risk of being excluded from public school. Two local philanthropists agreed to provide start-up funds for the first year of the program. The budget for the entire program, which included a four-week residential camp program for fifteen youngsters, a year-round mentoring program, parent counseling, and school consultation, was $10,000.

On that warm June day the two of us huddled together to figure out how to articulate the program's philosophy to the twenty new staff members inside the lodge. In our orientation, we had covered the basics: who were the children the program would be serving, what activities would be provided, what did the camp hope to accomplish. As we approached the end of the training session, one of the staff asked if any guiding principles or fundamental rules had been established for the program. As soon as the question was asked, we realized there had been a gap in our planning. We gave the new recruits a break and retreated to the side of the lodge for an executive session.

The framework established that day for the Bridge Program was not sophisticated. The conciseness of the guiding principles enabled the leadership of the program to communicate clearly with the staff and, in hindsight, probably established a precedent of simplicity that guided the program during its eight years of operation.

Driven by the pressures of time and a clarity of vision that sometimes comes from a sense of urgency, we agreed that staff should be guided by only two basic principles:

1. Ensure that children receive as many positive experiences as possible.
2. Keep the environment safe for all members of the camp community.

The creation of this program philosophy statement, a seemingly minor incident spawned by the practical necessity of the moment, was prophetic in several ways. The substance of the philosophy—creating opportunities for positive experience and protecting the well-being of children and staff—proved to be resilient. During its eight years of operation, the program continued to be guided by these fundamental principles. Not only did the content of the guiding principles prove to have enduring significance, but the manner in which that decision was made established a precedent for how the program would respond to the changing demands of the environment. Throughout its existence, the Bridge Program was characterized by (1) planning based on the needs of the children and families being served, (2) decision making that relied heavily on input from those affected by the decisions, and (3) an overall approach to challenges and opportunities characterized by flexibility and responsiveness. As the program evolved, staff came to believe that it was more important to recognize and learn from shortcomings than to be content with the status quo even when the current situation was perceived to be generally satisfactory. Their actions were guided by the image "If it's not broken but you can make it work better, then fix it."

The First Summer

Although short in length, the initial camp session was intense for all participants. Some children had never spent any time outside an urban setting. The campsite, with its thousand acres of unspoiled nature, evoked both pleasure and fear. The children enjoyed playing in the water and exploring the woods, but when night fell many of them became frightened by the darkness punctuated only by the sounds of insects and other creatures of the night. The attention given to them by staff was also unique for the majority of children. Many thrived on the interpersonal stimulation. For some, the stimulation filled an unmet need and allowed them to open themselves to the experiences of the camp program. For others, the attention was confusing and overwhelming. These youngsters either withdrew or rebelled against the personal attention they received.

The structured approach to programming was also unique for most of the children. Counselors were trained to plan activities with specific purposes based on children's needs and interests. Clear behavioral expectations were established, including rewards for compliance with and consequences for violation of rules that had been established to ensure positive experiences and to maintain safety—the original principles we established during training. As expected, many individuals tested the limits by consistently challenging these rules. One little boy with a low tolerance for frustration was prone to responding with a temper tantrum whenever he was confronted with a stressful situation. At times, he would strike out at other children and staff. His counselors handled the situation by providing opportunities for him to let off steam. They encouraged him to find a comfortable way to vent his feelings, such as taking a walk or punching his pillow. At the same time, staff encouraged him to talk about what was happening and let him know that they would work with him to resolve such situations. This child, who was accustomed to being spanked when he had a tantrum, did not know how to respond and, initially, escalated his acting-out behavior. Over time, the child learned that he was able to successfully manage his feelings without hurting himself or others. Like this little boy, most children at camp eventually responded favorably to the message that developing one's own internal control was preferable to having authority figures serve as external control agents.

The experience for staff was equally intense. Camp staff had a wide range of educational and life experiences. There was an exceptionally mature sixteen-year-old high school student and a sixty-year-old grandmother whose nurturing style more than made up for her lack of formal training. Several child-serving professionals came to the camp to get a break from the stilted environments in which they usually worked. A large number of undergraduate and graduate students who saw the camp program as a laboratory where they could apply their academic knowledge also participated. Even for those individuals who normally worked with troubled children, the intensity of spending twenty-four hours a day in an emotionally intense environment, with few creature comforts and little opportunity for privacy, tested their coping skills. Just as the children were asked to develop new ways to deal with stress and frustration, camp staff were also challenged to examine their traditional response patterns and to learn new approaches when their behaviors proved to be ineffectual.

By the end of the camp session, staff observed many changes in individuals as well as in the group as a whole. The majority of children demonstrated significant growth in communication and problem-solving skills. Their span of interest increased, and they appeared to be more self-assured. Some children seemed to be no different than they had been when the program began. In a few instances, children's functioning appeared to deteriorate. Most of the counseling staff reported having a very positive experience. Several students said that the camp program had solidified their commitment to pursuing a career in child services; others reported significant personal growth. It was a common perception among supervisors that staff actually benefitted more from the camp experience than did the children.

The change in the group dynamic was equally striking. Over the course of the camp session, the adults and children who participated evolved from a heterogeneous group of unconnected individuals to a fairly tight-knit community with a shared purpose. While predictable personality conflicts arose between specific individuals, on the whole relationships were positive and constructive. Without the pressures and distractions found in the city, where most participants lived, the energy of both children and adults was more readily focused on the development of facilitative relationships within peer groups as well as between staff and campers. Individuals—both adults and children—seemed willing to look at their own behavior and explore new ways of relating to each other. In addition to facilitating the achievement of therapeutic goals, this openness produced considerable personal growth and gratification. While it is possible to attribute many of these changes to the therapeutic techniques utilized in the camp program, most participants believe this growth was enhanced considerably by the power of an intense and positive therapeutic community.

When it was time to leave the camp setting, many tears were shed by children and adults. The realization that the support and camaraderie of the camp were ending, coupled with anxiety about reentering the complex and sometimes unsafe communities in which they lived, had a strong psychological impact on members of the camp community. For some, the grieving process extended well into the fall.

Life After Camp

After the camp experience, staff and children were eager to reconnect with each other, and arrangements were made for that to happen. Each child was assigned a counselor or a mentor, usually someone they had worked with at camp. Counselors met with children on a weekly basis to further develop their relationships and provide support and assistance in dealing with the children's issues and concerns. A parent counseling program was conducted by supervisory staff who often met with parents in their homes and other neighborhood settings as opposed to the traditional office-based approach. Liaisons were also set up with each child's school to assist teachers in applying what Bridge Program staff had learned about the children to the school setting and to provide intervention during crisis periods.

The positive halo of the summer program survived for a while. Unfortunately, the complexities of life and the inability to sustain the intensity of the camp setting eventually dampened the enthusiasm of those involved with the program. While some children maintained gains they had made at camp, others began to regress. A number of staff became discouraged and frustrated with their inability to sustain what had been achieved at camp. Some of this disillusionment was directly related to the loss of the supportive community that existed at camp. There were, however, other external factors that contributed to the dampening of positive feeling. At camp, some counselors did not have sufficient appreciation of the difficult environments in which the children lived. Poverty, neglect and abuse, and a general lack of stimulation and attention characterized the home environments for many of the children. In addition, staff came to recognize the limitations of the program's efforts to help the child. In many instances, the services, while well intended, did not have sufficient impact to make a difference.

Frustrated by these problems, we convened a planning retreat for the purpose of reviewing the program's past efforts and planning for the future. All staff were invited to attend, and a sizeable number actually participated. The planning session began with a review of staff's perceptions of the strengths of the program as well as areas that needed improvement. After hearing a variety of specific complaints and concerns, the group concluded that each component of the program was valuable, but within the current structure the program elements, individually and collectively, were not potent enough to achieve the overall goals of the Bridge Program. Ironically, the program, which had gone to great lengths to provide an alternative approach to the prevalent service delivery system with its bureaucratic, fragmented orientation, had inadvertently replicated some of the negative features of traditional approaches. Because of communication problems among the multiple individuals working with the children, families, and schools, and the absence of a holistic approach for responding to families, many of the children's needs were not being adequately addressed. Staff also became aware of the limitations of the service approach. Although from the beginning the Bridge Program recognized the importance of providing service to parents as well as to the identified children, in many situations there were other family members who required assistance. This was particularly true of younger siblings whose problems had not yet fully developed but who were clearly at risk of encountering difficulties at home, in school, and in other parts of the community.

During the planning retreat, staff eloquently expressed these concerns and struggled with the question of how to best address them. By the end of the session, the group had drawn three fundamental conclusions:

1.   Each family participating in the program should have a specific staff member assigned as the primary liaison. This individual would be responsible for communicating with children, parents, schools, and other organizations

and persons involved with that family. This person, who would be known as a Family Advocate, would be responsible for managing and integrating all aspects of the service program.

2. The scope of the Bridge Program should be expanded to include all children in the family as well as all aspects of family functioning that impact those children.

3. Restricting the program's role to providing direct service to a small group of families severely limits its impact. The program should explore ways to expand its scope in order to increase the number of children and families it could help.

By developing the role of Family Advocate and extending the focus of the program to the entire family unit, the Bridge Program was able to improve its efficiency and effectiveness. Through its nontraditional method of responding to families' needs, in whatever form they manifested, the program broke dramatically from the typical human services approach of narrowly defining specific domains of responsibility. This approach not only enhanced the program's ability to meet family needs, it also increased its credibility. At one point, a family's house burned down, and people in the Bridge Program were instrumental in finding them shelter and clothing and taking care of the children. The feedback received from family and community was very positive; here was a program that cared enough about the family to provide services in a flexible and sometimes very nontraditional way.

The role of the Family Advocate was complex. This individual was responsible for both direct service for children and families as well as system-focused preventive activities. These system interventions were directed at enhancing the ability of individuals and organizations to work more effectively with children at risk of or actually experiencing emotional and behavioral problems. Many of the system-oriented functions of the Family Advocate were carried out through educational and training activities. Internally, the Family Advocates were responsible for training and supervising counselors who worked at the summer camp program and the year-round follow-up. Externally, Family Advocates provided community education by conducting inservice courses and offering consultation to direct service providers and administrators in educational and social service agencies. Family Advocates also developed curriculum, conducted parent education groups for community agencies, and participated in local mental health planning efforts.

These external functions had been chosen for several reasons. Staff had considered increasing the number of families enrolled in the program. After considerable discussion, the group decided to limit expansion to a small number of families. Staff at all levels were concerned that if the program were enlarged many of the unique features of the Bridge Program community might be lost. They feared that if the program became much larger, the openness and flexibility of the program would be replaced by a more formal, rigid structure.

Having ruled out expanding the number of families to be served directly, staff explored other approaches. If they could not serve more families directly, then they would work with those individuals and groups in the community who had the greatest potential of positively influencing the development of children and families. This indirect or systems approach was adopted as a framework for developing the external activities of the program.

Because the Bridge Program adhered to the principle of tailoring services to the specific needs of the individual and family, the scope and nature of direct services provided by the family advocate varied from family to family as well as within a particular family over the course of involvement in the program. A critical component of the advocate-family relationship was a contract that defined the expectations, goals, and responsibilities of each party. This contract was typically written to encompass a short period of time with the understanding that it would be continually evaluated or renegotiated. The contract was viewed as a vehicle for solidifying the advocates' and parents' commitment to the process, in addition to spelling out the details of their activities. The following is an example of a contract between a single parent and her advocate (Apter et al., 1978):

ADVOCATE'S CONTACT WITH MRS. R

What Mrs. R. will do:

1. Meet with the advocate weekly and allow M to see his counselor weekly.
2. Keep a list of every bad behavior M does. (This was an attempt to get Mrs. R. to specify what annoyed her instead of thinking of her child as totally "bad.")
3. Begin to explore the possibility of beauty school. (Mrs. R. had reported that if given a choice she would like to be off welfare and be a hairdresser. Together, she and the advocate got information about schools, funding, etc., and she did enroll.)

What the Family Advocate will do:

1. Get a counselor to meet with M weekly, enroll him in Bridge Camp, supervise counselors who work with him.

2. Meet with Mrs. R. weekly to help her talk about and deal with her frustration with M and help her meet some of her own needs.
3. Be available to Mrs. R. in time of emergency or crisis. Be a support person in ways Mrs. R. can define.
4. Coordinate efforts of school and agency personnel working with the R. family.

The incorporation of these two major reforms—a preventive and ecological approach and the implementation of the family advocacy model—had a significant impact on the program's functioning. The inclusion of siblings and expansion of the scope of service to include indirect functions such as consultation and education greatly expanded the number of children and families affected by the program. The introduction of the family advocacy role, with its emphasis on coordination and integration of services, enabled the program to respond more effectively and efficiently to a wide range of family needs. A follow-up study, conducted by an independent evaluator (Apter et al., 1978), found that in a sample of thirty families that had been involved in the program during the course of its eight years, twenty-six children were still in school. In the sample taken since the beginning of the family advocacy program, all ten children were functioning in regular school programs. Both families and school personnel stated they had a much clearer understanding of the Bridge Program's role and goals since the family advocacy model had been implemented.

Given its limited budget and resources, the Bridge Program seemed to have a positive impact on the families it served as well as on the broader community. This does not mean that the program was without problems. As in most human services endeavors, the gains made by some children diminished once their participation ended. The uncomplicated, personalized approach of the program might be viewed as overly simplistic and technologically deficient in today's sophisticated environment. The program functioned in an era in which diagnostic and statistical manuals did not exist. There was little appreciation of or use of psychotropic medication. Nor was there much reliance on any of the state-of-the-art therapeutic interventions that are prevalent today, such as cognitive behavioral therapy. In spite of the Bridge Program's relatively simplistic approach—some might say because of it—the program made a difference in the lives of families. The emphasis on positive communication, a willingness to respond flexibly to emerging needs, and the comprehensive integrative role of the Family Advocate produced tangible gains in the behavior of the children and the quality of life for their families.

The Bridge Program Closes

In 1978, after eight years of operation, the Bridge Program ceased to provide services. Funding from a five-year Federal Demonstration Project Grant had expired. As with many demonstration projects, the promise of continued funding from community agencies did not materialize. The leadership of the program was weary from the intensive effort required to sustain the program and the cumulative economic stress caused by the low wages the program could afford. Most felt the need to move on to other endeavors. Ironically, at the time the Bridge Program was closing the reputation of the program was soaring within the community. The number of referrals from schools had risen significantly during the program's final years. Agencies were requesting training and consultation services from Bridge Program staff. Undergraduate and graduate students trained at the Bridge Program were bringing its philosophy into agencies for whom they were now working.

Did the Bridge Program represent an idea whose time had not yet come? Is it the nature of innovative programs to function so intensely as to drain themselves of energy within a short period of time? Did we devote too much attention to the substance of the program and not enough to building an enduring structure? While it is difficult to answer these questions definitively, one thing is clear: The Bridge Program's approach to serving families would not disappear with the closing of the program.

NOW

In the thirty years since the Bridge Program developed the family advocacy model, much has changed in the field of child and family services. Technology, in its multiple forms, has flourished. We now have a broad array of treatment and service interventions, and the burgeoning use of electronic data processing systems has radically altered the nature of communication in human services as well as all other aspects of modern life. The shift in political orientation has also had a significant impact. The growing distrust of government-operated programs and the concomitant movement to privatize services has not only shifted the locus of service delivery; it has also altered the quantity and quality of these services. Because human services, especially for the disadvantaged, have traditionally been associated with government sponsorship, the negative attitude toward government has translated into a reduction of public support for these service programs. In spite of President Ronald Reagan's rhetoric about the creation of a safety net, there is substantial evidence that fewer persons in need are being served and those who are being served are receiving less service (Himmelstein, Woolhandler, and Wolfe, 1992; Joe, 1984; Stoesz and Karger,

1996). Finally, the strong interest in containing costs and enhancing accountability has been translated into significant redesign of the manner in which services are delivered and paid for. Although these efforts to restructure service planning, provision, authorization, and financing have been most visible in the field of health care, recently care and cost management strategies have found their way into other human services sectors.

The degree to which these changes have impacted the manner in which human services organizations function is not debatable. A more interesting and difficult question is how have these changes affected the quality of services people receive and have these changes produced more positive outcomes. The focus of attention in this chapter is limited to one aspect of this complex set of questions. How have the multiple changes that have occurred during the past thirty years influenced the ability of human services entities to provide services that are responsive to the needs of families? Have the conceptual and technological reforms enhanced our ability to provide responsive, holistic, family-friendly services, or have these changes had no effect, or even worse a negative effect, on the lives of families who have sought help from the human services system?

Like most questions in this field there are no simple answers.

Managed Care and Families

The impact of using managed care strategies illustrates this point. During the initial stages of managed care, the primary focus is typically on controlling costs by reducing benefits and limiting access to services, especially those that are relatively expensive. These strategies are usually introduced in response to the perception that high-end services are being overutilized without producing positive outcomes. While managed care organizations have clearly demonstrated that cost and service utilization can be reduced by limiting benefits or requiring prior authorization before consumers are allowed access to services, these interventions certainly are not family friendly. By introducing a system of accountability that relies on measuring and controlling the number of units of service received, this strategy reinforces a problem-specific, fragmented approach to responding to family need. In addition, the use of external, third-party decision makers is inconsistent with an empowerment strategy that encourages families to be involved in determining how to best meet their needs.

It is interesting to contrast this managed care approach to the Bridge Program. Both operated within a framework of limited resources and a shared goal of providing necessary services in the least restrictive setting. However, the manner in which they related to families and the subsequent responses of consumers were markedly different.

On the other hand, more sophisticated managed care approaches, usually found in communities that have reached a higher level of service management and development, often incorporate principles of preventive and holistic service delivery while at the same time recognizing the importance of retaining consumer choice. In such systems, a single service provider agency may be given responsibility for all aspects of a family's health and well-being. A critical feature of this approach is to ensure that financial incentives are aligned with program principles and goals. Providers are often given a fixed amount of money for each individual or population. Assuming that controls are put in place to ensure that consumer needs are not being neglected—an assumption that is not always valid—it makes programmatic and fiscal sense for providers to focus on the preventive aspects of care. If the well-being of individuals and families is maintained and problems are detected and resolved early, providers will not be forced to utilize more intensive, high-cost services later on. Of course, this approach works only if those responsible for providing service are not able to abrogate their responsibility by shifting their financial liability onto other providers.

In more sophisticated health or social maintenance systems, consumers are able to choose their service providers. In such situations, providers are highly motivated to be responsive to consumer needs. In fact, measures of consumer satisfaction are often included in program evaluation packages.

Welfare Reform and Families

Welfare reform represents another major shift in human services policy and practice. The primary goals of this movement are to reduce the dependency of economically disadvantaged individuals on government subsidies and to promote employment and economic self-sufficiency among this population. While few would disagree that the welfare efforts of the past several decades have been unsuccessful, there is considerable disagreement about whether current initiatives will achieve their economic empowerment goals or will merely increase the number of poor people who do not receive welfare benefits.

As we have discussed throughout this book, perspectives on how to best improve human services are typically influenced by multiple factors that include political and philosophical biases, economic considerations, and the manner in which an individual's or group's vested interests will be impacted by alternative outcomes. The debate about welfare reform is no exception. At the heart of the controversy are differences in belief about the fundamental reasons that people remain on welfare. At one end of the continuum are those who believe that the open-ended nature of traditional welfare benefits serves as a disincentive for people to work toward economic and social self-sufficiency. Even those with a more liberal perspective recognize that many current welfare programs are economically punitive to persons who move from welfare to work situations. In many instances these individuals lose health benefits and are forced to assume the additional costs of child care and other services even though their income from employment is no greater than their welfare benefits. Conservative proponents of welfare reform believe that many welfare recipients have become accustomed to being taken care of; they believe that if the dependency option is removed, the current recipients will enter the workforce, albeit reluctantly. Persons holding this view also resent the fact that their hard-earned tax dollars are being spent by government on people who are "unwilling" to work for a living. Sometimes this resentment comes from lower-middle-class individuals whose income may not be much higher than that of welfare recipients.

Individuals who believe that the welfare program is merely a symptom of more fundamental problems in our society represent the other end of this continuum. This group believes that welfare reform must be approached in a comprehensive and systemic manner. Attention needs to be given to providing welfare recipients with skills that will enable them to enter meaningful career tracks rather than dead-end entry-level jobs. Proponents of this view believe that in addition to focusing on welfare recipients, attention should also be given to employers and other community institutions that may offer recipients opportunities to enhance their self-sufficiency. This belief is based on the premise that long-standing patterns of discrimination and rejection have demoralized many welfare recipients. Without a fundamental change in the receptivity of these institutions, it will be difficult to interrupt the negative cycle in which individuals who are economically disadvantaged, particularly ethnic minorities, experience rejection, lose their will to seek meaningful employment, and reinforce the public's perception that they would rather remain on welfare than work.

The systemic approach to welfare reform places a strong emphasis on providing supports necessary for an individual to prepare for and successfully enter employment while also ensuring that other critical family needs are being met. Welfare reform initiatives that focus on these systemic functions recognize the importance of addressing the individual within the context of his or her family. How these programs respond to family needs will determine their effectiveness in this domain. It is too early in the evolution of welfare reform to answer the question of whether organizations responsible for implementing these initiatives will be able to incorporate into their practice the principles of family-centered services described earlier in this chapter. Isolated examples of family-friendly approaches exist within welfare reform (Adams and Krauth, 1995); however, at this time these practices are not prevalent.

In some ways the dynamics of managed care and welfare reform are similar. However, at least one fundamental difference is likely to influence the extent to which these large-scale reforms will produce family-centered services. Managed health care is directed at a wide spectrum of individuals from all socioeconomic groups. Payment for health services comes from a variety of sources, including individual consumers, employers, and government agencies. Welfare reform, on the other hand, is directed exclusively at individuals in lower socioeconomic groups and is paid for almost entirely by governmental agencies that receive their support from taxpayers. This difference in clientele and funding arrangements influences how consumers are perceived and treated. As we noted in Chapter 2, agencies whose clients are viewed as irresponsible and intractable are less likely to receive support (Hargrove and Glidewell, 1990). Participants in managed care programs are more likely to be viewed as "paying customers" and therefore will be more likely to be served in a family-friendly manner. Welfare recipients are not as likely to fare so well. Those responsible for designing and providing welfare services consider the taxpayers, whose overriding goal is to move current recipients from the welfare rolls, to be paying, ultimately, for the program. Because of these funding dynamics, welfare recipients are less likely to be viewed as customers whose preferences and needs should be considered when services are being provided.

Reinventing Family Advocacy

As we have seen from the examples of managed health care and welfare reform, the current agenda for human services is ambitious and complex. Reconciling political, economic, and programmatic forces that vie to shape today's human services programs is no easy task. Given the traditionally compartmentalized and fragmented nature of human services, coordination of function and goals represents a formidable challenge. The utilization-management initiative of the Comprehensive Services Act for At Risk Youth and Family (described in Chapter 10) illustrates the difficulties inherent in developing family-centered services within the current human services environment characterized by fiscal constraint and increased emphasis on accountability. Even though the legislation and program philosophy of the Comprehensive Services Act provide an excellent framework for serving children in a family and community context, the political, fiscal, and organizational dynamics make it difficult to actualize this concept.

The dilemma is, in part, a workload issue. Juggling these multiple demands is itself an enormous task. There is, however, another dimension to this dilemma. The strategies necessary to enhance accountability—specifically, fiscal and utilization management—are in some ways diametrically opposed to the underlying principles of family-centered services. (In simple terms, a fundamental conflict exists between bean-counting techniques, which are essentially reductionistic, and a systems-oriented approach to service delivery that stresses the importance of understanding and supporting the connections among individuals, functions, and organizations.) A case manager operating under an accounting system that quantifies care into specific units of service, each of which has a predetermined cost, will find it difficult to gain approval for a holistic, family-centered service plan. Conversely, a managed care organization requiring providers to justify activity in terms of individual diagnostic and functional criteria for various levels of service may have trouble appreciating the value of indirect services given to families on behalf of an identified client.

The task of reconciling these various and sometimes competing goals and directions is difficult but not impossible. Having a sufficient understanding of the multiple forces that are impacting policy and practice is helpful. Knowing that many of these dynamics are cyclical in nature may also make it easier to understand and adapt to the current demands of the environment.

Let us apply this perspective to the subject of family-centered services. One might ask why the Bridge Program in the 1970s, with its scarce resources, was able to develop a comprehensive approach to family services that was consistent with the principles and values of holistic, family-centered care. Yet twenty-five years later, with considerably more knowledge and sophistication within the field of human services, we are still struggling with the challenge of how to effectively integrate services in response to the multiple needs of the children and families we serve. Ironically, at the time the Bridge Program operated conditions may have been more favorable for the development of a cohesive family-centered approach. Vestiges of the activist, community orientation of the 1960s still existed during that period. What the Bridge Program lacked in financial resources and technological sophistication it made up for in the simplicity and flexibility of its organization. Layers of administrative bureaucracy were minimal, and the channels of communication were open within the program as well as between the staff and the families they served. In the ensuing thirty years, the United States has undergone a significant shift in its political and social orientation. These changes, which were in part a reaction against the ambitious liberal orientation of the 1960s, were also shaped by the growing awareness of limited resources and a strong conviction that human services organizations needed to be held accountable for their performance. As the philosophical pendulum shifted further in the direction of a businesslike approach to human services, many individuals realized the shortcomings of an overly reductionistic approach. The response to this recognition has been a reintroduction of more holistic, ecologically oriented approaches and an increased emphasis on customer satisfaction. Thus, a family-centered orientation appears to be reemerging.

How this approach will evolve and what it will look like when it is more fully developed is unclear. The added complexities of today's environment make it unlikely that the next version of family-centered services will closely resemble the family advocacy model of the Bridge Program. There is, however, a high degree of probability that the emerging approach to serving families will share many of the basic concepts and values found in the family advocacy approach that enjoyed a brief period of recognition and success nearly three decades ago.

POINTS TO PONDER

1. The Bridge Program was created in an environment that is quite different from the one we live in today. What are some of the issues that developers of family-centered services face today that did not have a significant impact in the 1970s? What strategies might be used to deal with these issues in trying to create a service system that is truly responsive to family needs?

2. Identify a situation in which you or a member of your family were a consumer of human services. Assess the extent to which this experience was family-friendly. What were the factors that made it responsive to the needs of your family? What were the factors that made it seem unresponsive to your family?

3. One of the points made in this chapter is that the way in which staff of the human services organization are treated will affect the manner in which they will relate to consumers of the services they provide. How would you design a staff's supervision and support structure to enhance their responsiveness to the needs of individuals and families?

4. What are the primary political and social forces of the late 1990s that might support or impede development of family-centered services?

CLASSROOM TO COMMUNITY

Applying the Concepts of Change

- From your readings, develop a list of questions that will help you differentiate between services programs that are responsive to families and those that are not. Using these questions, interview several persons who are involved in various aspects of the same service program, such as provider, administrator, direct consumer, family member. Identify major differences and perspectives. Discuss what accounts for these differences and what might be done to reduce the differences in their perspectives.

- Familiarize yourself with a retail store or other business endeavor that has a reputation for providing exemplary customer service. Through observation, interviewing, and reading, identify the characteristics of this business organization that contribute to its success in satisfying customers. Include policies and practices among these characteristics, as well as other aspects of the organization that make it customer friendly. Discuss how a human services organization might draw upon its business counterpart to improve its consumer-friendly relationships. Are there features of this business organization that you would not wish to transfer to an organization that is concerned with providing human services?

4

OPENING THE GATES
Making a Children's Psychiatric Hospital More Responsive

*I'm not a psychologist, but . . . if you have any sort of organization,
a business—any sort of an endeavor where there are a lot of people
involved, change is always difficult.*

~ George Allen, Governor of Virgina

I n accordance with the principle of inertia, an institution will remain at
rest or continue on the same course unless acted upon by an external
force. Simply altering the speed or direction of an institution does not,
however, ensure that the service it provides will improve. Constructive
change requires repositioning an organization in relation to its external
environment, such as consumers, other service providers, and funding
agencies, as well as reorienting and preparing members of the organization
to effectively manage and cope with the changes. In this chapter we describe
the process of integrating a public children's psychiatric hospital into the
broader community. We also present strategies employed for refocusing the
hospital's mission and program to be in line with community needs.
Finally, we discuss how the leadership of the hospital worked with staff to
help them adapt to these changes and function more effectively.

In the summer of 1984, I stepped down from my lofty position as Associate Commissioner in the New York State Office of Mental Health and became director of the Virginia Treatment Center for Children, a small state-operated psychiatric hospital for children and adolescents in Richmond, Virginia. I had spent the previous six years immersed in the complexities of service delivery systems, policy analysis, and funding mechanisms. Although I had received an excellent education about how mental health services were planned, regulated, and managed at the state level, and had become painfully aware of how political forces shaped the state's efforts to respond to human needs, I was ready for a change.

The position in Virginia would certainly be different. Directing a hospital would put me much closer to the everyday reality of providing services for young people with serious emotional problems. It would also give me an opportunity to put into practice the ideas and strategies I had accumulated during my twenty years of experience in the field of child mental health. What made the position particularly attractive is that the person who hired me, the commissioner of mental health in Virginia, wanted someone to play a leadership role in the development of child mental health services for the Commonwealth as well as to direct its best known children's facility.

It was an exciting challenge, and I was looking forward to becoming more directly involved in the day-to-day reality of working with people at the community level. There was only one potential problem: Would my free-wheeling, open-ended style be compatible with the highly structured, institutional culture of the hospital?

This was a question I would struggle with during my first months at the treatment center—and for the next fifteen years of my tenure as director.

At times I will refer specifically to my own perceptions and actions in relation to the hospital. However, it should be noted that for the most part, the changes that have evolved at the hospital are the product of a team effort, with staff members as well as families, personnel from a variety of child-serving agencies, and other concerned citizens contributing to the development of a program responsive to community and family needs.

SETTING A NEW COURSE

Initial Impressions

I spent the first month in my new position meeting with staff from the hospital, representatives of agencies that interacted with the hospital, and other individuals interested in child mental health services in the Richmond area. I wanted to understand how the treatment center was perceived, its strengths and problems, the manner in which it cared for children, and its relationship with the community. At the completion of this process, I was overloaded with information and bewildered by the wide-ranging and often conflicting views of the treatment center. The only consistent theme was the negative perception of the hospital by external parties—people from academic, community service, and state government settings. While acknowledging that staff of the treatment center were intelligent and well-trained, individuals interviewed felt that the hospital underutilized its resources, did not serve children and adolescents in greatest need, and did not fulfill its research mission. Community providers viewed the treatment center as a country club, selecting only those patients who were good candidates for trainees to observe and work with, rather than admitting children based on the intensity of their needs.State officials perceived the treatment center as trying to distance itself from its public service mission; and academics bemoaned the lack of research productivity. Each group tended to view the treatment center's deficits in relation to its own interests.

A sense of fragmentation and isolation existed within the hospital. Each department believed it was working hard to care for children and adolescents but did not have the support or assistance of other departments. When employees of the treatment center learned that the community perceived them as elitist and unresponsive to the needs of children and families, they were genuinely surprised since staff viewed themselves as dedicated mental health professionals. Staff acknowledged that the absence of a permanent director for the past five years had taken its toll, leaving the center without a clear sense of direction and purpose. In spite of this lack of leadership, staff continued to work diligently to provide treatment and care for those youngsters who were admitted to the hospital.

As I tried to put together these diverse and disparate perceptions, I came to several conclusions:

1. The hospital had suffered, both in its internal functioning and its community relations, during the prolonged period without stable leadership.

2. The problems of the hospital stemmed not so much from a lack of staff competence and dedication as from organizational adaptation to aversive conditions. In response to the lack of internal direction, staff had acted self-protectively, erecting barriers between themselves and other departments to fend off criticism and encroachment.

3. In the absence of internal leadership and clear, unified direction from external organizations such as the state department of mental health and the university, the treatment center had become disconnected, dysfunctional, and limited in its productivity.

4. The treatment center needed a renewed sense of purpose, a clear set of long-and short-term goals and objectives, and a detailed plan of action to guide the hospital back to a role of prominence and leadership within the child mental health system of the Commonwealth.

5. Finally, I realized that even if I had the wisdom of Solomon and the patience of Job, my efforts would be doomed to failure unless the new course set for the treatment center was one that was supported by the major constituency groups associated with the hospital. Given the hospital's lack of clear direction, the provider and academic communities' pervasive negative perceptions of the treatment center and the sense of isolation experienced within the hospital, any course of action was unlikely to be viable unless it addressed the child mental health community's major concerns and came from a credible source that represented the interests of all of the constituent groups.

A Road Less Traveled

Arriving at these conclusions was not too difficult. Deciding what to do next was not as easy. After some deliberation I decided that the next logical step would be to develop a plan of action to guide the treatment center toward a productive leadership role within the child mental health system. This decision brought into focus my first critical choice. While my preferred style of organizational operation was to directly involve persons responsible for performing the work in deciding what should be done, that did not seem to be a viable alternative in this instance. I decided instead to turn to the outside, the external environment, and I convened a program review committee comprised of individuals from a variety of settings, who had a strong common commitment to child mental health.

After consultation with the commissioner and chief of staff of the Department of Mental Health, thirteen prominent professionals and citizens were invited to participate in a committee charged with formulating a purpose and plan of action that would enable the treatment center to effectively carry out its mission within the child mental health system. The group, which was comprised of public and private mental health practitioners; a parent of a former patient at the treatment center; faculty from psychiatry, pediatrics, and nursing; a member of the state board of mental health and mental retardation; and representatives from education, court services, and mental health agencies at the local and state level met for three months to develop a set of recommendations for the future direction of the treatment center. The committee was asked to address two questions:

1. What are the most critical child and adolescent mental health needs and problems in the Commonwealth of Virginia?
2. Within its current resource base, what should the treatment center do to most effectively respond to these needs and problems?

The broad, open-ended wording was designed to encourage the review committee to consider the role of the treatment center within the context of its broad mission of research, training, and service delivery rather than simply focusing on immediate, direct service needs. This emphasis was intentionally chosen because of the absence of a clear direction and systematic approach to addressing child and adolescent mental health needs at the state level.

Under the leadership of the director of a private psychiatric hospital for children and adolescents in Richmond and the executive director of a community services board in northern Virginia, the committee conducted a systematic review of current studies and statistical information about mental illness in children and adolescents in the Commonwealth as well as the treatment center's patient services, staffing, and funding. The committee concluded that the treatment center, with the largest pool of expertise in child mental health in the state, should play a vital role in providing treatment, training, and research on behalf of children, adolescents, and their families in Virginia—a role that no other organization was performing. The committee recommended that the treatment center play a leadership role in building an integrated child and adolescent mental health network comprised of practitioners, academics, and other individuals or organizations concerned with the mental health of children and adolescents and their families. Essentially, the committee envisioned the treatment center as the hub of two interlocking sectors—service providers and university faculty—in order to facilitate the development and dissemination of knowledge and skills. The goal of these activities was to enable service providers to work together effectively to provide comprehensive, holistic services for children and their families. The committee recognized that the absence of adequate policy, funding, and management for child and adolescent mental health in the Commonwealth had a negative impact on the treatment center's ability to fulfill its mission, and the committee encouraged the state to take steps to remedy these problems. The committee offered the following specific recommendations for the treatment center:

• The treatment center should continue to strive to fulfill its role in child and adolescent mental health services by providing a balance of services, research, and training activities.

• The center must develop close liaison and coordination with the department of psychiatry at the medical college, the community service boards responsible for mental health services at the local level, and other agencies and facilities in the public and private sectors that are concerned with delivery of child and adolescent mental health services, training, and research.

• There should be a well-defined administrative structure that clearly describes the roles, responsibilities, and relationships of the treatment center and other key organizations within the integrated system. The treatment center and the local community services boards should develop an agreement describing criteria and procedures for planning and implementation of mission, treatment, and discharge planning of patients that will be built on principles of accessibility, availability, appropriateness, and quality of care.

• The treatment center should concentrate on providing intensive services at the inpatient and partial hospital level, with the community services boards taking primary responsibility for outpatient services.

• A medical/clinical director should be hired and jointly supported by the department of psychiatry at the medical school and the treatment center.

• The treatment center should expand and strengthen its training services and programs by hiring a training director and developing comprehensive training opportunities both within the center and for agencies and facilities concerned with child and adolescent mental health.

• The treatment center should develop a viable research program that will have statewide relevance through the hiring of a director of research as well as in the development of a major leadership role in research of state-of-the-art technology and treatment of children who are experiencing serious mental illness.

The program review report was unanimously endorsed by the committee and was presented to the commissioner of the state department of mental health, who accepted the recommendations and directed us to implement them.

CREATING NEW CONNECTIONS

The program review committee's report provided the hospital with a blueprint for establishing the treatment center as a resource center for the child and adolescent mental health services system within the region. After reviewing the report with staff of the hospital, we began the process of realigning internal operations of the treatment center and creating mutual interdependence among the major parties involved in the child and adolescent mental health system. One of the first steps taken was to renegotiate the relationship with the department of psychiatry of the medical school. The chair of the department of psychiatry, who had served on the review committee and was supportive of the plan to link the academic and public sectors, agreed to jointly fund a faculty position within the treatment center. The child psychiatrist occupying this position would have the dual functions of serving as chair of the division of child psychiatry and medical/clinical director of the treatment center. The chair of psychiatry also agreed to establish a faculty position for the director of research, which would also be partially funded by the university. This unprecedented investment of resources and commitment to public child mental health services established a firm foundation for strengthening the quality of service, training, and research provided by the treatment center.

At the same time, a small team from the treatment center began to work with the local community services boards to establish formal agreements defining the respective roles and responsibilities for all parties. A group of hospital and community providers met on a regular basis and within several months had drafted a memorandum of agreement that essentially transferred some of the basic gatekeeping functions, such as admissions decisions, from hospital to community services board staff. In return, community providers agreed to become involved in treatment and discharge planning at the time of the child's admission. The agreement also underscored the importance of involving the child's family, as well as related service agencies such as education, social services, and juvenile justice, in these planning activities. The establishment of these agreements was made easier by the state department of mental health's recently issued policy on prescreening of hospital patients. The policy directed local community services boards or their designees to screen for appropriateness all individuals being considered for admission to public state-operated psychiatric hospitals. The complementary nature of the state policy and the local agencies' abilities to negotiate this agreement demonstrates the importance of having higher-level support for changes at a local level.

Having established an external structure for working collaboratively with the academic and community provider sectors, the next step was to attend to the internal functioning of the hospital. The prolonged absence of permanent stable hospital leadership had taken its toll on the staff. Within the hospital a "fortress" mentality had developed, with staff isolating themselves from the external community as well as other segments of the hospital organization. Direct communication between individuals was rare, and when it did occur it was often critical or defensive in nature. The reactive, protective mode of interaction among staff was further exacerbated by the absence of clear expectations and boundaries. The relationships among professional disciplines were characterized by concern with status within the hospital hierarchy and territorial disputes rather than cooperation and collaboration.

Despite the insulated, divisive work environment within the hospital, the majority of the staff continued to demonstrate an exceptional degree of dedication and compassion toward the children and adolescents served by the facility. This strong commitment to young people with serious emotional disturbance appeared to provide a common bond that kept the organization intact and, in limited ways, productive, in spite of staff responses to each other and to the community. Recognizing that staff's dedication to children was a strong asset upon which to build more effective programs, we established a multipronged plan to realign the internal operation of the treatment center to be compatible with the family and community orientation developed by the review committee. This plan included the following objectives and activities:

1. *Develop a leadership team that would reflect the mission and functional organization of the hospital.*   At the time the review committee issued its report, the executive committee was comprised of the director, acting medical director, and assistant director for administration. The assistant director for administration took early retirement and the acting medical director, who had served as acting director of the hospital for a year, expressed a desire to return to his role as clinical practitioner and educator. The executive committee was reconstituted to include the director of training and director of research as well as medical director, assistant director of administration, and director. The first priority was to hire a medical director who would also serve as chair of the division of child psychiatry in the department of psychiatry of the medical school. We were fortunate to be able to hire a child psychiatrist whose clinical philosophy included a strong family and community focus and who had an interest in actively promoting research and training related to clinical practice. A director of training, with considerable experience in working with mental health services and community agencies, was also hired. The final position on the executive team, director of research, was not filled for several years.

2. *Reorient clinical philosophy and practice to be more family and community oriented.*   We recognized that the shift in treatment approach would take time to accomplish and required structural changes in the pattern of service delivery as well as intensive education of staff.

The revised clinical approach was based on several assumptions:

- Children and adolescents should be admitted to a hospital level of care only when they cannot be treated safely at the less restrictive level.
- The objectives of hospital level of care should be limited to dealing with those problems and issues that made it necessary to remove the child from the home setting. Legitimate functions of hospital treatment include stabilization of the child, assessment of strengths and needs of child and family, and collaborative planning for post-hospital service and care.
- Hospital activities should be conducted jointly with families and community agencies. The locus of responsibility for child and family situations should always remain with family and community.
- Unless strong and continuous efforts are made to maintain the hospital as an open system, there will be a powerful tendency for the institution to revert to an insulated, exclusionary status.

Based on these assumptions, we initiated a number of actions designed to educate staff and realign organizational structure in the direction of being more responsive to child, family, and community needs. These initiatives included the following:

1. *Offering staff an alternative perspective.*   It is not possible to introduce significant change in a complex organization, such as a psychiatric hospital, without making a significant investment in staff education. We brought to the hospital a number of training programs conducted by persons who had actually designed and delivered short-term, focused hospitalization programs that involved families. With the help of treatment center staff with expertise in family systems approaches, we designed our own multisession training program to help staff reorient their approach to children and families. We were careful to ensure that all staff, including direct care and support service staff, were involved in these educational activities.

2. *Alteration of treatment delivery patterns.*   We were fortunate that many of the organizational changes required to develop an interdisciplinary team approach had been undertaken previously. The inpatient unit had been organized into two age-specific units, each having its own dedicated staff of mental health professionals. The nursing department had established a primary nurse system in which each child was assigned a specific nurse who had responsibility for all aspects of his or her nursing care program. Each team

also had a designated psychiatrist, psychologist, social worker, occupational therapist, recreational therapist, and nutrition specialist.

Nonetheless, there were significant structural impediments that made it difficult to shift to a more responsive, inclusive approach to providing treatment. As is the case with most child mental health agencies, a clear division of clinical labor existed. A psychiatrist was always responsible for medication management; the child had his or her own therapist, sometimes someone other than the individual dealing with medication; another professional provided family contact and therapy; and a social worker typically dealt with community agencies. This segmented approach fostered fragmentation and inefficiency, made communication difficult, and usually left families and communities in a state of confusion. The absence of clear definition of roles and responsibilities for discipline departments such as psychiatry, psychology, and social work and clinical units such as children's inpatient units further exacerbated the disjointed treatment process.

To remedy this situation we clarified and realigned roles within clinical staff. Shortly after his arrival, the medical/clinical director introduced the single therapist approach, assigning one professional staff member to be responsible for all aspects of a child's treatment, including individual and family therapy and liaison with community agencies. This consolidation of roles not only increased efficiency of communication but also enabled the therapist to have a more comprehensive, holistic view of the child and family situation and facilitated family and community involvement in treatment planning and delivery.

3. *Improving communication and conflict resolution.* We also took steps to enhance the functioning and coordination of disciplines and departments. A small committee, comprised of a cross section of staff from the hospital, was convened to define the roles and responsibilities of individuals, departments, and units. Committee members were also asked to develop a clear process for encouraging constructive communication and problem solving. One of the committee's most significant contributions was to clearly delineate the roles and boundaries of clinical service units such as the child inpatient program and professional discipline departments. Basing its recommendation on the assumption that clinical decisions should be made at a level closest to the actual day-to-day interaction with children, the committee proposed that primary responsibility for clinical decisions and treatment be given to clinical units. Professional discipline departments were given the responsibility for providing staff selection, training, and supervision needed to ensure that the

services being delivered by members of their disciplines met the highest professional standards. While this matrix arrangement was still complex, designating specific points of responsibility and accountability for clinical decision making and quality assurance eliminated much of the organizational confusion and bickering that existed prior to clarification.

At the level of individual functioning, the committee developed a set of guidelines for dealing with communication among staff. The basic underlying principle of the committee's recommendation was that direct communication was the most effective means of resolution. If an individual had a concern or problem with another individual, then those persons should speak directly to each other. If those individuals could not resolve the issue, either because of irreconcilable conflict or an absence of knowledge, then the issue would be brought to the next level in the supervisory hierarchy. This chain would continue until it was satisfactorily resolved or was arbitrated by the highest appropriate level in the organization. Final authority for clinical matters resided with the medical/clinical director. The director of the hospital would be the last arbitrator for other issues.

4. *Strengthening the supervisory process.*   Once the decision-making and communication guidelines were finalized, we turned our attention to putting these principles into practice. We chose the management supervision process as the primary vehicle for implementing our new policies. Supervision was defined broadly to include the provision of clarification, assistance, and support that staff needed to perform their jobs effectively, as well as the traditional supervisory functions of monitoring and evaluation. Expectations for supervisory behavior were established, including the right of each employee to have a scheduled, face-to-face meeting with his or her supervisor no less frequently than every other week and preferably once a week. In these sessions, supervisors were expected to clarify work expectations, review performance, and engage in mutual problem-solving activities with the supervisee. Supervisors were also asked to provide constructive feedback and offer assistance to the employee in improving work performance. Since most human services managers have not received formal management training, we decided to offer a four-session inservice course on how to develop an effective supervisory program.

Building an Effective Child Mental Health Constituency

As the hospital organization became more productive in fulfilling its service, training, and research missions, it became apparent that the goals we had established could only be fully accomplished with the assistance of other groups and organizations. Two gaps became obvious. First, it was difficult to have an effective partnership with families without an external organization dedicated to the development and support of families. Second, the hospital, as a service provider organization, had only limited credibility and potency in advocating for improved child mental health services. Experience had demonstrated that the most effective advocates were citizen groups representing a wide spectrum of community interest and perspectives. We decided to take an active role in facilitating the establishment of family and citizen groups that would work with us to promote the development of a responsive system of child mental health services.

In the spring of 1985 the treatment center sponsored a conference on developing partnerships between parents of children with serious emotional disturbance and professionals. Among the 300 participants at the forum were a number of parents who had children in the child mental health system. With the assistance of the patient advocate of the treatment center, a small group of these family members began to meet to discuss how they could form a parent support and advocacy group. In a few months the Parents and Children Coping Together (PACCT) group was established. (This group has since expanded from a small informal group of parents who met several times a month in a conference room at the treatment center to a statewide organization with twenty-four chapters and several hundred members. In addition to the valuable role this group has played in advocating for improved services for their children, PACCT has also served as a valuable resource for educating and supporting families who have been admitted to the treatment center. New families are routinely referred to PACCT upon admission so they might receive support and learn from other parents how to navigate the complex child-serving systems.)

Shortly after the PACCT group was formed, we decided to establish a citizen advisory council for the treatment center. Unlike many advisory groups, this council was designed to have a broad educational mission. Rather than confining its focus to supporting the hospital, the council adopted an expansive vision of increasing awareness of, and advocating on behalf of, children's mental health. The council, comprised of professionals and lay persons interested in improving services for children and families, adopted the following mission and goals:

1. To educate and inform the general public and service providers on mental health issues affecting children and families and on services and gaps in service for these children and their families.

2. To educate and train a variety of professionals and students in children's and family mental health issues, including the following:
   Residents and medical students in various specialties
   Students and trainees in mental health-related disciplines
   Professionals who must deal with these children
   Judges, attorneys, and related professionals
3. To identify and advocate in the legislative and executive branches for adequate programs and resources for public mental health services and for parity in private programs.
4. To support research in childhood mental illness.
5. To raise funds on behalf of mental health programs for children.
6. To develop coalitions with other groups concerned with children's mental health issues.
7. To stay informed regarding the Virginia Treatment Center for Children and advise when appropriate.
8. To support volunteer efforts at the treatment center.
9. To inform the general public about the treatment center.

While the primary focus of the council was on the broader mental health system, we also suspected, based on prior experience, that there might be a time when the council would need to advocate on behalf of the treatment center. Unfortunately, several years later this premonition proved valid when the state department of mental health decided to close the treatment center in response to the state's fiscal crisis. Largely because of the advisory council's efforts, the governor reversed this decision. Without the advisory council's quick and effective mobilization of support, the treatment center would have been closed in spite of its demonstrated excellence in service delivery, training, and research. (Chapter 5 describes how the hospital coped with the threat of closure and subsequent events.)

Another positive achievement of the advisory council was its role in promoting the development of a comprehensive, integrated system of care for children and adolescents with serious emotional and behavioral disturbance and their families. Under the leadership of the woman who was then first lady of Virginia and served as honorary chair of the advisory council, an interagency forum convened involving cabinet secretaries and agency heads, legislators, service providers, and advocates. The purpose of the conference was to develop a plan for promoting interagency collaboration. This forum led to a series of other initiatives on behalf of troubled children and their families, and it eventually culminated in the enactment of the Comprehensive Services Act for At Risk Youth and Families in 1993. This legislation created an organizational and funding structure that enabled localities to develop individualized, locally based services for troubled children and their families with an emphasis on family involvement.

A WORK IN PROGRESS

A number of exciting changes occurred during the first few years of the hospital's transformation. The new partnership with community providers improved communication and led to more effective coordination of services for children and families. Most community services boards designated a single liaison person for children. These liaisons served as the primary point of contact and coordinated the child and adolescent activities within their agencies. The liaisons for the larger service boards visited the treatment center on a regularly scheduled basis and were given office space so they might meet with therapists to discuss children from their agencies who were being treated at the hospital. Our targeted approach to dealing with the problems that caused the child to be admitted to the hospital rather than focusing on all the child's needs, and the increased coordination with families and community agencies, had an impact on the duration of hospitalization. The average length of inpatient stay declined from more than five months in 1986 to forty-five days in 1989 and fifteen days in 1993. This reduced length of stay enabled us to see many more children with the number of admissions increasing eightfold over a nine-year period.

As the hospital's relationship with community agencies improved and collaborative efforts expanded beyond services provided by the hospital, we began to work cooperatively with other groups to improve the continuum of care available in the community. A number of joint proposals for service enhancement were developed by the hospital and community agencies. One striking example of the role of the hospital as a facilitator of change was the development of a therapeutic foster-care program for two nine-year-old boys who had spent significant portions of their lives in psychiatric hospitals and other institutional settings. At the time the program was developed, both boys had spent prolonged periods of time on the children's inpatient unit at the treatment center because the community had been unable to find alternative placements. Their history of aggressive behavior had even caused several residential treatment centers to refuse to consider the boys for placement, even though the locality was willing to pay the annual fee of more than $100,000 per child. With the relatively rapid turnover of other children at the hospital, the boys became demoralized, which led to an escalation of their disruptive behavior. While the local community was committed to helping these boys, typical agency territoriality and bureaucratic fragmentation prevented the agencies from effectively coordinating the development of a suitable program for these children.

Confronted with what appeared to be a hopeless situation—having the boys relegated to a highly restrictive hospital program for an indefinite period of time—the leadership of the treatment center approached the community agencies with an appealing offer. The treatment center proposed to establish an intensive therapeutic foster-care program in the local community. Hospital staff would take responsibility for designing the program, recruiting foster parents and ancillary staff, and providing respite and emergency services during the initial phase of the program. The boys would remain in the hospital until the program was fully developed, with a transition phase in which the children would continue to use some aspects of the hospital program as they gradually moved to full community placement.

The only obligation of the community agencies—public schools, community service boards, and social services—would be to provide funding for the foster parents and ancillary staff and to arrange for transportation to the public school when the children were prepared to attend. At the end of the development phase—slated for six months—the city would assume operation or responsibility for the program.

This bold proposal, with an associated cost of less than 25 percent of what the city would have to pay for placement in a residential treatment center, motivated the local agencies to accept the offer and work together to develop a fiscal and operational plan to support the initiative.

There was considerable skepticism about the program during its initial phase. Staff at the treatment center who had seen the high level of aggression of these two boys were not very confident that they could be managed in such a nonrestrictive setting. Community agency personnel were understandably anxious about the risks of personal injury and property damage. In spite of this wariness, the program succeeded. By the end of six months the boys were fully integrated into their foster homes and were attending the local public schools. The local child-caring agencies assumed responsibility for the program with the local community services boards serving as the lead agencies. The therapeutic foster-care program quickly expanded to serve additional children and, at this date, is still in operation.

While this program did not result in reuniting the boys with their biological parents—both of the boys' mothers had been uninvolved and inaccessible for several years—the collaboration between hospital and community agencies not only succeeded in creating a homelike setting for the boys, but it also expanded the expectations and perceptions of hospital and agency staff in regard to development of individualized, community-based service programs for children with serious emotional and behavioral disturbance.

Enhancing Family Involvement

One of the most tangible results of the reorientation of the hospital program was the increased presence of families within the hospital setting. The inpatient units expanded visiting hours and adopted a more proactive approach toward parents. In order to make them more comfortable in the hospital setting as well as to encourage the exchange of information about the children's needs and behavior, family members were invited to participate with their children and unit staff. In a few instances, parents with young children who lived some distance from the hospital were invited to stay on the units with their children for periods of up to ten days. Although gaps were still noticeable in the hospital's responsiveness to families, especially in relation to arranging for clinical services to be available at times that were most convenient for families, a noticeable increase occurred in the inclusion of parents and other relatives in the planning and delivery of services.

Strengthening Research and Training Programs

During the period in which clinical services were being reoriented toward families and community, staff also became involved in providing training in response to expressed community needs. In some instances, treatment center staff provided educational programs directed at enhancing knowledge about understanding and treating children with serious emotional problems. In other cases, the treatment center invited nationally recognized educators to conduct training on state-of-the-art approaches such as developing in-home programs and case management services. In addition to providing seminars and workshops, the treatment center also initiated a monograph series directed at supplying providers and parents with easy-to-understand summaries of what is known about clinical topics relevant for child and adolescent mental health. Individuals familiar with research in a particular area were commissioned to write forty- to fifty-page monographs on subjects such as child and adolescent suicide, responding to aggressive behavior, and sexual abuse of children. These monographs were distributed to local mental health agencies, other child-caring agencies, and individuals interested in learning more about child and family issues.

At the same time, the treatment center began to develop its own research base, with an emphasis on studies that would enhance our understanding of the service delivery process. A director of research was hired. A number of small pilot studies were conducted, and planning was initiated to develop a research and clinical database for the hospital that would serve as a major source of information for treatment planning and research.

The problems of developing research and training programs within a clinical hospital setting soon became apparent. With a limited pool of personnel and money, and constant demand for clinical services, it was difficult to mobilize sufficient resources to conduct research and training activities even though the hospital had committed a small portion of its budget for these purposes. In response to this dilemma, the executive committee of the hospital decided to establish a specific entity exclusively dedicated to research and knowledge dissemination activities. In the winter of 1989, the Commonwealth Institute for Child and Family Studies was created as the research and training branch of the treatment center. Established with the blessing of the commissioner of the state department of mental health and the chair of the department of psychiatry at the medical school, the institute served as a locus for research and training, enhancing the visibility and value of these activities within and outside the hospital while also providing a small measure of protection for these functions. The institute drew upon the expertise of staff and faculty at the hospital as well as individuals from other academic settings, community agencies, and family organizations.

IN CONCLUSION

This chapter describes how a public psychiatric hospital for children and adolescents evolved through direct service, research, and training from a self-contained, isolated institution to a proactive multipurpose center working in partnership with families and community agencies to better serve families with children and adolescents with emotional problems. During this protracted process of organizational change, the hospital has been viewed as a subsystem within the broader child-caring community, which includes, among others, families, child-serving agencies, and academic programs. The integration of the hospital with other components of the child-caring community has been guided, in part, by the following ecological concepts.

Position
- For an organization to be responsive to family and community needs it must occupy a central position within the system. At the time of our initial assessment, the hospital described in this chapter was clearly in an isolated, peripheral position in relation to these other subsystems. During the six-year period covered in this chapter, the treatment center moved to a more central

position, exerting more interests on the other components of the system and, in turn, becoming more susceptible to the actions of other members of the child-caring network.

Boundaries

• The degree to which organizational boundaries are open has a significant impact on the ease of communication and movement between subsystems. Increasing the permeability of the boundaries between the treatment center and the other subsystems was an important component of the change process.

• Opening the boundaries of this organization involved dual efforts: initiating outreach activities from within the hospital as well as inviting external groups to become more involved in hospital activities.

Stability

• Organizations may range from being rigidly fixed in a single pattern to being in constant flux. At either extreme, an organization's functioning may be severely hampered. Organizations with rigid, routinized patterns of operation do not have the flexibility to adapt to the constant changes that are occurring in our current environment. On the other hand, an organization in constant flux is forced to devote most of its effort to coping with change, leaving it with little time or energy for its service mission. Effective organizations tend to shift along a narrower band within the stability/flux continuum. In the case of the treatment center, the organization was initially relatively stable in spite of the negative perceptions of surrounding constituent groups.

Locus of Intervention

• Since no immediate external impetus for change existed at the treatment center, staff had little motivation to alter the agency's fixed pattern of functioning. Therefore, it was necessary to enlist the assistance of people and organizations outside of the hospital to create momentum for change. (As you will see in Chapter 5, when a strong external force poses a serious threat to the integrity of an organization, internally initiated adaptation is more likely to occur once individuals within the organization recognize the need for change.)

Balance

• According to an ecological/systems approach, an organizational subsystem is constantly in the process of adjusting or adapting to reach new equilibrium. Long-term constancy is neither desirable nor realistic. A change in one subsystem impacts other subsystems, which in turn further affects the original subsystem. Organizations, like other organisms, undergo a cyclical and evolutionary process of development, working through successive stages of differentiation, integration, redifferentiation. During the six-year period described in this chapter, the treatment center and its staff experienced considerable change. While the changes were generally viewed by most as positive, it was also clear that the organization could benefit from a period of equilibrium. Unfortunately, this was not to be the case due to externally driven events (described in Chapter 5).

POINTS TO PONDER

1. The initial change in direction for the hospital relied heavily upon direction from the external environment. How would Hersey and Blanchard's situational leadership model (Hersey and Blanchard, 1969, 1996) view this approach in light of the status of the hospital at that time? What other strategies, if any, do you believe might have been utilized to effectively achieve change?

2. In the process of restructuring the hospital's program, considerable attention was given to establishing a framework and processes to enhance staff communication. Does this approach have relevance to a human services organization you know? How would you intervene to improve staff interaction in this situation?

3. In an era of scarce resources, human services organizations are increasingly forced to establish priorities. The treatment center attempted to establish a balance between responding to a small group of children whose needs required intensive intervention and focusing on enhancing the knowledge and capacity of the broader community through research, training, and consultation. What guiding principles, if any, should organizations consider in trying to establish an appropriate balance? What is your assessment of the treatment center's approach to this issue?

4. One of the most difficult aspects of organizational change is modifying the culture in which staff are accustomed to functioning. In a hospital or other self-contained institutional setting, breaking down the barriers between facilities and the internal and external environments, such as between families and community agencies, is especially difficult. What strategies did the treatment center employ to make the staff culture more responsive to the external environment? What other approaches might have been effective for this purpose?

CLASSROOM TO COMMUNITY

Applying the Concepts of Change

- Select an institution that is currently undergoing change. Through observation and interviews, identify major threats that these changes pose to persons involved with the institution. What are the principal factors underlying this concern or fear about change? Discuss alternative approaches to reducing resistance and increasing acceptance of the proposed changes.

CHAPTER 5

STANDING AT THE PRECIPICE
Coping with the Threatened Closure of a
Children's Facility

It is best to stay alive, alert, trust yourself, but not give up, no matter what the situation is. Get in there, stay in there, figure it out, but don't look back.

~ Natalie Goldberg, Writer

How does a human services organization cope with the impending th reat of closure? What are the issues that leadership and staff have to deal with, and what strategies do they employ in response to external political forces and internal staff and organizational dynamics in order to effectively deal with the crisis while maintaining, as much as possible, business as usual? The following chapter illustrates how a psychiatric hospital used the principles of leadership and balance to cope with the threat of closure.

~

The day before Labor Day weekend 1990, the commissioner of the state department of mental health called a special meeting of the department's executive staff and facility directors. He provided us with an overview of the state's unanticipated $2 billion budget deficit. He explained how each agency had been given an expense reduction target and had been asked to develop a plan for meeting its revised budget goal. He described a series of actions the department would take to consolidate programs and streamline support services. He told us the decisions had been difficult and painful, but that in order to reach the budget target substantial reductions were required. Rather than making large across-the-board cuts, an action that might jeopardize all services, he had chosen to eliminate several programs and, in one instance, an entire facility, in order to achieve the necessary savings.

Then he announced that as of January 1, 1991, the Virginia Treatment Center for Children would no longer operate within its current building. Instead, the budget would be reduced by half and the remaining staff would be reassigned to the child and adolescent units of the two large state-operated psychiatric facilities in the Central Virginia region. The goal of this realignment, he explained, was to take the strengths of the existing program and "transfer" them to the other facilities. While there may have been a theoretically logical rationale for this realignment plan, it was obvious to me, and I suspect everyone else in the room, that implementation of this plan would effectively put the treatment center out of business.

It would not be an overstatement to say that my reaction to this news was similar to that which one experiences when told about the death of a close friend who had been in perfect health. The treatment center was generally considered to be the best child psychiatric facility in the state. We had recently been cited by the Joint Commission on Accreditation of Health Care Organizations as being in the top 10 percent of all facilities surveyed. We had a staff of distinguished and dedicated professionals and direct care staff whose diagnostic acumen and therapeutic skill were frequently applauded by families and community agencies we served. We had been nominated for— and subsequently received—a prestigious significant achievement award from the Division of Hospital and Community Psychiatry of the American Psychiatric Association. The State Department of Mental Health, Mental Retardation, and Substance Abuse Services, the agency that had decided to close our program, had recently bestowed upon us its State Human Rights Program Award for a therapeutic foster-care program we had developed with the city of Richmond. With our long history of quality service and the positive perception by the community, how could this be happening to the treatment center?

As I struggled with my confusion and numbness, another painful realization emerged. The news of our demise, which would be announced at the state board the next morning, would soon become public information. It was critical that staff at the treatment center be made aware of the decision before they heard about it through the rumor mill or the media.

And once everyone knew, what then? Should we simply line up like good civil servants and evacuate the building at the designated time, leaving behind our program that we had worked so hard to develop and the children and families we served? Or should we refuse to accept the wisdom of his decision and attempt to alter what appeared to be a programmatically unsound, but nonetheless inevitable, course of events?

Returning to the treatment center, I struggled with these questions. My limited repertoire of experience did not contain many relevant precedents, and I certainly did not have enough time to develop a systematic plan. By the time I reached the hospital, I had developed a brief list of people I needed to inform immediately, and I had made one critical decision: There was no way I could accept the decision to close the hospital without trying to save it.

BREAKING THE NEWS

I met with the executive committee of the hospital to discuss strategies for informing staff. We decided to hold a series of meetings the next day to allow us to reach everyone who worked at the hospital. We began with the management team and then held three other meetings to ensure that all staff could attend. With its twenty-four-hours-a-day operational mode, the hospital presented a formidable challenge for providing accurate and complete communication. Since the executive committee had adopted the position that staff should have all available information, it was particularly critical to communicate directly with the entire staff in a short span of time.

Facing the staff on the day before the Labor Day weekend was a difficult task. I had delivered bad news to them before, but not of the magnitude of that day's message. After describing the department's decision and plan as well as the rationale behind them, I wanted to present some suggestions to help staff cope with the multiple stresses and demands that lay ahead. I decided to frame this guidance in the form of a set of expectations: what I expected of myself and what I expected of the staff. I began by enumerating my expectations for the staff during this crisis period. I said that I expected them to do the following:

- Maintain patient care in a professional manner
- Support other staff during these difficult times
- Understand the distinction between their roles as staff members and as private citizens

The latter expectation was intended to assist them in addressing the dilemma of being both state employees and citizens of the Commonwealth. As state employees, staff were prohibited from engaging in political activities such as legislative advocacy. As citizens, on their own time, they certainly had the right to voice their opinions. It is a fine line but one with clear rules and boundaries.

After addressing what I wanted from staff, I turned to what I expected of myself. I stated that I would do the following:

- Give them complete and timely information on what was happening regardless of whether the news was good or bad
- Work to find the best alternatives for preserving the core values and services of the hospital
- Make the transition as smooth as possible for patients and families if the transfer were to actually occur
- Be available to help staff in any way possible during these difficult times

After I had completed my statement, I asked if there were any questions or comments. The glazed eyes and lack of response seemed to be good indicators that the staff were in shock.

During the next few weeks we held meetings for the entire staff on almost a daily basis. The initial reaction of shock was soon replaced by an outpouring of intense emotions, including frustration, anger, and fear. We worked hard to fulfill our promise of keeping staff informed, and, in spite of the impending loss and future uncertainty not only of the program but also of each individual's employment status, the hospital continued to operate smoothly. I received numerous messages of appreciation from staff for our efforts to keep them informed, and the common crisis we were experiencing seemed to bring everyone together, creating greater cohesiveness than there had been prior to the crisis.

Our constant emphasis on maintaining high standards of patient care seemed to serve several purposes. First, it provided staff with a tangible focal point for their energies, allowing them to channel their intense feelings into useful activity while also serving as a distraction from a traumatic situation over which they had little control. Second, with the personal demoralization and loss of self-esteem that naturally accompanies such a devastating loss, staff were able to salvage some sense of pride by being able to continue their roles as helpers for the children and families who came to the treatment center in dire need of assistance. Finally, given even a remote possibility the treatment center would be saved, we knew that any drop in vigilance and dedication by the staff would lead to deterioration in the quality of service, making it difficult to regain the previous standard of excellence, even if the program survived. Thus, our concerted effort to maintain a positive work environment served multiple personal and programmatic functions.

GETTING READY TO FIGHT

The treatment center's advisory council (described in Chapter 4) had been established for several purposes. The major goals of the council were to provide a broad-based forum for addressing child mental health issues through public education and advocacy and to support the hospital by procuring modest sums of money for equipment and activities that were not covered by the operating budget. However, another unstated purpose guided the establishment of the council.

When I worked in the New York State mental health system, I watched other programs, some of them exemplary, struggle with program reduction and consolidation decisions driven by budgetary and political considerations. In some instances, good programs simply disappeared. In other cases, decisions were altered and programs were "rescued." The critical survival factor for vulnerable agencies appeared to be the presence of an articulate, assertive constituency group that was able to persuade decision makers that it was in their best interest to maintain the program. While it seemed unfair that program decisions were so heavily influenced by political consideration, the reality was that decisions to cut budgets were often political rather than programmatic. Following the axiom that political bodies will often take the path of least resistance, constituent advocacy was a potent tool for preserving effective human services programs. Therefore, when the advisory council's membership was being determined, special attention was given to ensuring that such strong advocacy groups as the Mental Health Association and the Virginia Federation of Women's Clubs were sufficiently represented.

As we had hoped, the advisory council responded rapidly when told of the impending closure. An emergency session was called and members of the council developed an action plan to mobilize support for the treatment center. Several thousand letters were sent to individuals interested in child mental health services, informing them of the problem and asking them to contact legislators and the governor. Individuals who had personal relationships with policy makers were asked to make direct contact. A contingency of the council met with the leadership of the department of mental health and the secretary of health and human services to explore alternative resolutions to the budget crisis. An aggressive media campaign was mounted, including convening a press conference in which members of the advisory council described the devastating impact of proposed cuts, including the closure of the treatment center, on children's services in the Commonwealth.

The immediate objective of this campaign was to make the governor and legislators aware of the negative effect this budget reduction strategy would have on services for children with serious emotional disturbances and their families. By calling attention to the problem, the council hoped to stimulate discussion about alternative solutions. Members of the council recognized the serious nature of the state's fiscal shortfall. They did not want to downplay the significance of the financial crisis but wanted instead to promote exploration of alternative strategies that would not be as harmful to the children's service delivery system. Their campaign was intended to ensure that the treatment center issue remained visible while alternative scenarios were being explored. In this regard, the advisory council was successful. The local newspaper, with its politically conservative editorial viewpoint, did not traditionally respond favorably to public human services issues. Yet the newspaper provided extensive coverage of the story and, much to our surprise and delight, even printed an editorial asking the governor to reconsider the decision to close the hospital. A member of the advisory council was told by a staff member of the executive branch that more letters and telephone calls were received by the governor's office about the closing of the treatment center than any other decision in the governor's $2 billion budget reduction plan.

One of the most ardent supporters of the treatment center was the chair of the department of psychiatry at the medical school. He was concerned about the impact of the service reduction, but he also anticipated that the reduction in education and research functions would have a serious adverse effect on the division of child psychiatry since the treatment center was the major training and research resource for the child and adolescent academic psychiatry program. Since the university was state supported, the chair was constrained by the same limitations on legislative advocacy as other state employees. He did, however, spend considerable time educating the advisory council about the importance of the treatment center and making other members of the mental health community aware of the problem. He also initiated conversations with the medical school administration regarding the possibility of incorporating the treatment center into the university.

After several weeks of intense activity, the first visible sign of progress appeared. The governor commented in a newspaper article concerning budget reductions that he was reconsidering the decision to close the treatment center. With this positive indication, efforts to find an alternative solution to the programmatic and fiscal problems were accelerated. Three options were identified:

1. The treatment center could remain within the mental health department in a downsized capacity to serve as a transitional facility for youngsters placed out of state who were being returned to their home communities by the social services department and the youth services division.
2. The hospital could be converted to an educational residential treatment center.
3. The treatment center could be transferred to the Medical College of Virginia of Virginia Commonwealth University.

Given the governor's willingness to reconsider the decision to close the hospital and the legislature's strong negative reaction to what they perceived as a unilateral policy decision made without their input, the leadership of the Department of Mental Health took an active role in exploring alternative arrangements. Discussions were held with the university administration as well as the commissioners of other state agencies to determine whether any of the proposed options were feasible.

Although the governor's announcement that he might reconsider the decision to close the treatment center created a sense of hope among its staff and supporters, considerable anxiety and tension still characterized the environment. Stress was exacerbated by the continuing preparation for the possible closing. Mock layoff-planning meetings were conducted with central office staff to identify individual staff members who would be affected by the closing. To make matters worse, the state personnel system contained employment protection provisions for those with greater seniority. If an individual's position were abolished, that person might then displace another individual who in turn would displace someone in a different position. This domino effect led to a pervasive sense of anxiety among all staff since, potentially, they might be impacted not only by the treatment center closure but also by other reductions of positions within the department.

In addition, relationships with the central office were strained. Staff from the department of mental health were less than pleasant in our interactions with them. I attributed this negative reaction to their displeasure about us challenging the decision to close the hospital. I found myself continually struggling with the conflict between fulfilling the duties of my position as a state employee and maintaining my loyalty and responsibility to the program, the families we served, and the staff of the center. Finding a balance between advocating on behalf of the treatment center and staying within the boundaries of organizational appropriateness was especially challenging. On the one hand, I believed that the services we were providing were valuable and would be significantly diminished under the plan proposed by the department. I had no ambivalence about the correctness of my position. On the other hand, Virginia's legal code explicitly prohibited state employees from lobbying legislators, and I felt a personal responsibility to respect the organizational chain of communication as long as I was employed by the state. I did not, however, feel obliged to remain passive while the treatment center program was being dismantled.

My resolution regarding this dilemma was to provide information and support to the treatment center's advisory council. This group, comprised of a cross section of citizens and incorporated as an independent, not-for-profit organization, was not restrained by the same rules as the employees of the hospital. Members of the advisory council were able to act assertively within the executive and legislative branches of government as well as to provide their perspective to the general public through the media.

Maintaining an appropriate balance between my role as a state employee and my commitment to the treatment center's program was not always easy. At times I was tempted to communicate my opinions to the policy makers more directly, but reason prevailed. In spite of my restraint, I was viewed by some within the department as disloyal and was, in one instance, accused by a state official of acting in a manner that could be construed as insubordinate. In spite of these difficulties, I generally felt comfortable playing a leadership role in maintaining productivity and the well-being of the hospital while serving in a consultative capacity to the advisory council.

DETAILS AT ELEVEN

If I was not prepared when I heard the announcement that the treatment center would be closed, I was equally surprised to hear, precisely four weeks after the initial announcement, that the decision had been changed. Late one afternoon I received a call from a newscaster from one of the local television stations asking if he could come to my office to interview me. When I asked what the subject was, he explained that the secretary of health and human services had announced before the state senate's finance committee that there would be a delay in closing the treatment center, perhaps indefinitely and at least until June, while alternative proposals were considered. I do not recall what I said in the interview, which aired on the evening news, but I am fairly certain that my comments, made in the midst of trying to process this new information, were not very coherent.

The next several months were as chaotic, but not as terrifying, as the first four weeks. In addition to being actively engaged in developing a viable plan for the treatment center's continuation, we also had to tend to the internal functioning of the hospital. We were dealing not only with the continuing uncertainty of the future but also coping with the aftereffects of the initial trauma. While staff were relieved and happy that the center would remain open, considerable uncertainty hung over the future, as well as a strong sense of loss. Even if the treatment center were to continue to function, it was clear that the hospital would not be the same as it had been before the threatened closure. Staff felt betrayed and abandoned by the parent organization, the state department of mental health, and the "near-death" experience had altered everyone's perspective. For many individuals, the shock of learning that their workplace would no longer exist had a debilitating effect, ranging from confusion and somatization to almost psychological paralysis. For others, the event shook them from their complacency, forcing them to come to terms with the tenuous nature of their work life, which they had previously taken for granted. A few individuals, realizing the treatment center would no longer enjoy the luxury of being fully subsidized by the state, decided to take a proactive role in shaping the future of the hospital. These individuals, some of whom had previously shown no inclination toward leadership, became strong advocates, promoting staff cohesiveness and working diligently to identify and perform the tasks required for ensuring the continued viability of the hospital.

During the next few months we continued to focus our attention on both external and internal environments. While the future administrative home of the treatment center was being negotiated, we were actively involved in helping people grieve the loss of their past work environment, celebrating a reversal of the decision to close the hospital, and preparing for the demands of the future. Staff of the hospital developed and implemented a number of coping activities. One of the most popular initiatives was a series of celebrationlike healing activities that were sponsored on a rotating basis by the departments in the hospital. One department prepared a special breakfast for staff, another unit developed a treatment plan for employees. Each week a special theme day was declared. Staff were asked to wear their favorite buttons or their most colorful T-shirts or to bring a small gift for another employee whose name had been drawn from a hat. Paradoxically, staff cohesiveness increased dramatically during this stressful period. Traditional territorial conflicts were set aside, trivial complaints were rarely heard in meeting rooms or corridors, and employees took time to listen to and provide support for other staff members.

Deliberations about the future of the treatment center continued through-out the fall. Many of the initial options failed to materialize because of lack of interest or resources and were discarded. Eventually, only one viable alter-native to closure remained: Our fate hinged on the willingness of the medical school and its hospital to assume the financial risk associated with incorpo-rating the treatment center into its administrative structure.

Finally, after several months of negotiation, an agreement was reached. The medical college hospital would assume full responsibility for operation of the treatment center. Programmatic, budgetary, and administrative authority would be transferred to the university. The department of mental health would, in return, provide a $1.5 million per year subsidy and would lease the building to the university for $100 per year. The university would retain all revenues collected but also would be responsible for any deficit beyond the $1.5 million. The university would provide assurance that the treatment cen-ter would continue to serve its traditional target population of medically indigent individuals and would maintain its close working relationship with the community services boards. The participating agencies signed a five-year agreement that included periodic evaluations of the new arrangement.

We breathed a collective sigh of relief and began to make preparations for the complex and difficult transition to our new home.

INGREDIENTS FOR A SUCCESSFUL RESCUE

What accounted for the successful outcome to this potentially disastrous sit-uation? Although no simple answers to this question can be found, several factors appeared to play a significant role in saving the treatment center. Obviously the quality of the program and its good reputation were assets. These attributes alone, however, were not sufficient given the severity of the fiscal crisis the state was experiencing. Consider the fate of the geriatric unit whose closure was not reversed. This program enjoyed an equally stellar rep-utation, yet it did not survive. The most obvious difference between the two programs was that the treatment center had prepared the groundwork for staving off threats to the integrity of its program by developing strong rela-tionships with the surrounding community, especially through the forma-tion of its advisory council. The support of the medical school's department of psychiatry and the interest and willingness of the university and its hospi-tal to "adopt" the treatment center were also key factors. The chair of the department of psychiatry, recognizing the importance of the child psychiatry program to the department's mission, advocated assertively on behalf of the treatment center.

As one might expect, however, programmatic value and good intentions are not sufficient driving forces, especially during periods of economic austerity. An additional fiscal factor contributed to the university's decision to "adopt" the treatment center: Many of the families we served were low income and, therefore, eligible for Medicaid coverage. In its effort to limit unnecessary utilization of psychiatric hospitals, the federal government had established restrictions on reimbursement for individuals admitted to state-operated and other free-standing psychiatric hospitals. States were allowed to tailor these restrictions to their own unique circumstances. Virginia, which had a large supply of private psychiatric hospitals for children, had decided to limit Medicaid reimbursement for juveniles to children and adolescents admitted to psychiatric units of general hospitals, of which there were very few. When the treatment center was operated by the department of mental health, it was considered a free-standing psychiatric hospital and was, therefore, not eligible for Medicaid reimbursement. By becoming a component of the medical college hospital, the treatment center's status was redefined. It was now considered to be a unit within a general hospital and, therefore, eligible for Medicaid reimbursement. With this additional source of revenue, the university projected a good possibility of breaking even financially.

The final element that may have contributed to the treatment center's success was less tangible. Staff at all levels had enormous pride in their work and were not willing to accept what they considered to be an unreasonable decision. At the same time, staff were sophisticated enough to understand the appropriate role they must play—or not play—within the rescue process. They were also resourceful enough to remain focused and cohesive during a period in which slippage in programmatic productivity might have produced irreparable damage to the quality of the program. The fact that the staff had just recently adjusted to significant changes in the programmatic direction of the hospital may have enhanced their resiliency to change.

IT'S NOT OVER EVEN WHEN IT'S OVER

The signing of the agreement to transfer the treatment center to the university was greeted with enormous relief and jubilation. After five months of anxiety and uncertainty, staff were delighted that the treatment center's future was secure, at least for the next few years. This period of celebration, however, was short-lived. Transferring the administrative oversight of the hospital from the department of mental health to the medical college hospital proved to be a daunting task. Staff not only had to become acquainted with a new group of personnel at the medical school hospital; they also had to become familiar with an entirely new set of regulations and procedures. Even though the department of mental health and the university were state agencies, most of the record-keeping and processing systems were different. Converting the clinical, administrative, and fiscal procedures to the university's required considerable effort. Even after the new systems were in place, it took staff a full year to become fully acclimated to the new procedures.

Psychologically, the adjustment was even more difficult for many staff members. While everyone was grateful to the medical college hospital for "adopting" the treatment center and staff at the new parent organization were cordial and supportive, establishing good working relationships was not always easy.

The stress of adjusting to a new administrative environment was compounded by the residual effects of the threatened closure experienced by many individuals. The shock of suddenly learning that their workplace might vanish, and the subsequent anxiety generated by the prolonged period of uncertainty, took its toll on everyone. In some instances, individuals went through the normal grieving process with its full range of accompanying emotions. Other individuals were more severely impacted, experiencing the same post-traumatic stress symptoms exhibited by the children we serve. Somatic distress, depression, and impaired functioning were not uncommon. For some staff, these problems persisted for several years. Even individuals who had risen to the challenge of dealing with the crisis often had delayed reactions as much as one or two years after the initial trauma.

On the positive side, the experience of surviving such a serious threat to the existence of the hospital helped to prepare staff for the accelerating pace of change. A few years later, the medical college hospital underwent a major reorientation and streamlining process in response to managed care pressures. Staff at the treatment center were appropriately concerned about the potential organizational and personal impact of the cost-reduction effort but were able to understand what needed to be done and to engage more quickly in constructive activity to address the problem than some of their coworkers in the larger hospital who had not personally experienced this type of crisis.

One of the lessons that may be gleaned from this near-closure experience is that traumatic change has an enduring impact on an organization as well as its members. Even when constructive coping strategies are utilized and a successful outcome is achieved, as in the case of the treatment center, the leadership of the agency needs to continually monitor the status of the program and staff. Continual clarification of the organization's mission, guiding principles, and programmatic direction will help to reduce confusion and misunderstanding. In light of the unstable nature of the contemporary human services environment, setting clear expectations and direction is particularly critical and should extend to the level of organizational and programmatic procedures to ensure that services are provided in an efficient and responsive manner. Finally, supervisors at all levels need to be sensitive to how staff are responding. In addition to monitoring for signs of post-traumatic reaction, it is important to adopt a proactive position toward employee morale. Helping staff cope with the additional stress produced by change is a cost-effective strategy that yields not only more satisfied employees but also more effective provision of services.

POINTS TO PONDER

1. Can you relate the near closure of the treatment center to anything you have experienced? How are those events similar or different?

2. From your readings, can you identify something that could have been done differently and better?

3. What relevance do the theories of leadership and organization described in Chapter 2 have for the hospital crisis described in this chapter?

4. In Chapter 2 we discussed how individuals who participate in the change process often experience this change as a loss. How were staff of the treatment center assisted in dealing with the grieving process? What other strategies might have been employed to help them deal with the threat of closure and subsequent events?

CLASSROOM TO COMMUNITY

Applying the Concepts of Change

- As part of the welfare reform initiative, the local welfare department has been told that welfare recipients cannot be on the rolls more than two years. Government officials project that with this program the number of people on the welfare rolls will be cut by 50 percent within the next two years. In keeping with the principles of total quality management, the local director has charged social workers in that department with coming up with a plan for how the department can adapt to meet this challenge. As members of this department, your responsibility is to develop this plan. The tasks you must accomplish are the following:

  - Identify the issues and functions that must be addressed in this plan, such as individual issues, organizational design, and programmatic content. Specify which internal and external forces must be addressed.

  - Describe the program, including the changed roles of workers needed to accomplish this goal.

  - Describe how you would manage issues such as reducing the size of the workforce and preparing remaining staff.

CHAPTER 6

STEPPING OUT
Moving from Campus to the Workplace

The price one pays for pursuing any profession, or calling, is an
intimate knowledge of its ugly side.

~ James Baldwin, Writer

M any factors, including age, race, and gender, shape the perspective of an individual working in any field. This chapter presents an account of a new college graduate entering the work of human services. Making the transition from academia to a full-time working life is difficult. This chapter examines some of the forces at work in a small nonprofit organization and the challenges and rewards this work offers to a young person.

~

ON CAMPUS: A 1990s PERSPECTIVE

In 1992 I attended my first large national political march with a group of women from the college I was attending. It was the first time that my abstract interest in activism was played out in such a large community effort. I had grown up listening to tales of marching on Washington and finally I was in the midst of thousands of people making their presence known to the nation.

The incredible surge of energy I experienced as we stopped in rest areas and shared the moment with travelers convinced me that these events would be part of my adult life. I was exhilarated by the sense of shared goals and interests. I had no idea how much more was required to form a functional community or movement.

In high school I had done quite a bit of volunteer work, most of which ceased in college because I was busy with my studies. I had started researching AIDS on my own, clipping every newspaper article I encountered and attending conferences. I had also been a member of an acting troupe whose goal was public education surrounding mental illness. My first year at college I made plans to start such a group on campus, but I could not find the time to organize the group.

My academic and social experiences in college might have led to a greater expectation of the complexity of organizations. Working in the relatively new and evolving field of women's studies provided a theoretical perspective on forming community and the issues that accompany this process. Concurrent to our classroom discussions of diversity, we were all witness to or participants in various campus struggles surrounding diversity of class, race, religion, and sexuality, to name the top contenders. To its credit, the college administration was making efforts to encourage civil dialogue. However, the college president, whose position required extreme diplomacy, seemed more concerned with the public image of the college than with the harmony of the student body.

The majority of my experiences within the college's organizations and communities were not negative. I was inspired to pursue work in human services by many positive experiences. Since my initial bus trip to march on Washington, I have attended many marches of celebration and protest. The act of marching, however, carries limited impact. At gay pride marches in New York City, I am both inspired by the sheer numbers and disappointed by the lack of action and energy. While visibility is important, an immense amount of work needs to be done.

In college, discussion often did generate satisfactory change. In this environment, individuals followed basic tenets of respect and listening. Though these parameters felt stifling at times, I learned quickly that I had been lucky to work in this environment. Many people outside academia did not, and still do not, find it necessary to play by such rules. However, all the talk often resulted in little action. I have found through my own experience and discussions with other young people that many undergraduate experiences do not provide the skills necessary to create real change or to cope with the waves of change that exist in the postcollegiate world.

ENTERING THE FIELD

Upon graduating I moved to New York City and began to explore jobs in publishing and the nonprofit sector. I decided the business of publishing was not for me, and I fell in love with a job opportunity in a transitional-living community for homeless mentally ill women. I wanted to dive into the task of saving the world, and I had a particular interest in working with mentally ill women. After two months of interviews and waiting, I was turned down for the job. I continued working as a temporary employee in a variety of offices and ultimately accepted a position as a fundraiser for a nonprofit law center serving nonprofit community organizations in low-income neighborhoods.

I was a little disappointed that I would not be providing direct services or doing advocacy work. However, I recognized that by writing grants and organizing mail appeals, I would enable the attorneys to provide direct services to clients. I held onto the notion that the job I had not gotten would have been the perfect position until some of my friends began similar jobs as program assistants for human services organizations. For us young people in the field, the majority of these positions were administrative by nature, the job titles meant very little, and in a way we were paying our dues. My experience was similar to that of many new graduates. We wanted to make a difference, and we did not understand the many forces that would affect our work within organizations.

My work in development began three weeks before a huge gala "friend-raiser" for the nonprofit organization and consisted of assembling "goodie bags" and managing the guest list. Before I wrote a single grant proposal I had "socialized" with several hundred funders, politicians, clients, and volunteers and had memorized most of their names from invitation lists. However, I hadn't actually spoken to any of these people. As a young woman quite new on the job, I was virtually ignored at this event. In some respect, I felt like I should have stayed behind the scenes. Many major players from business, law, philanthropy, and the nonprofit sectors were present, and there was a culture of recognition, mutual favors, and general politicking that left me on the outside. This feeling would resurface throughout my time with this organization. It was my first sense of the nonprofit sector being similar to the corporate world. Despite the progressive mission of the organization, its supporters—and hence the people with the influence—were primarily white male corporate attorneys.

I learned quite a lot about the importance of the mechanics of coordinating events. In fact, the success of fundraising in general relies heavily on minutiae.

During these first weeks my mission was clear, and I had no concept of the issues that would arise in the following months.

The organization for which I worked was in a tricky position in terms of gaining financial support. The organization receives no government funding, and nearly 40 percent of its funding comes from foundations. Philanthropic giving is tight, and there is not much room for growth or expansion of funding from foundations in the current climate. Furthermore, I worked for a group of attorneys. Despite the fact that these attorneys provided free legal services to low-income groups, fundraising for lawyers can be difficult. I learned very quickly that the image of the organization was as important as the actual work accomplished, especially in terms of gaining financial support.

I worked closely with a development consultant who had worked with a variety of nonprofit organizations. My explicit responsibilities included grant writing, reporting and compliance, and direct mail appeals. In truth, I was responsible for database maintenance, some clerical work, correspondence, and communications, all to some degree. In addition, because I was raised in the computer age and am computer savvy, I was called upon to answer technical questions for my coworkers.

Most of the people I worked with had been practicing nonprofit law for many years. In this realm, and later in others, I recognized the challenges presented by change. Though the demands and variety of these tasks excited me, I found myself being spread thin rather quickly.

A DELICATE BALANCE

I learned a great deal in this position about diplomacy as well as the mechanics of fundraising. In my naivete, I had no idea that politics within the organization had so much impact on fundraising. Many individuals are involved in the operations and funding of a nonprofit organization, and all of them must be satisfied with the outcome. When writing grant proposals or letters for mail appeals, I was presented with a dual challenge: to describe the work of the organization and to make it sound "sexy" enough to gain financial support. This challenge harkens back to the concept of market-driven organizations (see Chapter 2).

The executive director was very concerned that we achieve this goal of "sexiness." When describing the work of the organization I had to choose particularly high-impact, compelling cases. We worked with hundreds of nonprofit groups that were doing important work in education, art, social welfare, and community and economic development, but we focused repeatedly in our materials on four or five. Another aspect to our self-promotion was appropriate gratitude to our volunteer attorneys and funders. There were moments when it was easy for me to forget that we worked for a nonprofit organization since so much of our work involved corporations and huge law firms. We placed an advertisement in a well-known business publication, and I remember quite clearly the conversation that preceded the writing of the ad. The executive director, our consultant, and I met for a brainstorming session. We spent an hour trying to come up with a slogan to lead the advertisement, which would list our funders. Of course, the advertisement would thank them, but the true goal of the advertisement was to spread the word about the organization, hence drumming up more business and more funding. At such a moment it took great effort to remember that this process led to the access of resources by our clients and was not just a game of business and marketing.

I was fortunate enough to attend several meetings of the board of directors. In contrast to the board of the student alliance in college that I had observed, this group consisted of high-powered attorneys from top law firms, with a smattering of attorneys from nonprofits. The staff discussed the lack of racial diversity and community representation but concluded that the directors most capable of helping the organization were those at firms. An effort was made to recruit individuals of color. This group was well-organized, and most of the directors were genuinely interested and invested in the work of the organization. Nevertheless, most of the discussion focused on the financial health of the organization. The development staff, including me, reported to the group each meeting about the success of our fundraising, and most of the subsequent discussion about new initiatives for the organization centered around our concerns.

Within the office many people had their hands in the business of fundraising. In my position, I had to report to several people. I reported to the executive director primarily and then to the consultant. I was expected to work independently, but much of my work had to be reviewed or approved by another person before I could send it out the door to meet a deadline. The director and consultant were the only other persons responsible for fundraising. However, my work involved describing the accomplishments and goals of every individual in the organization. Each person, with his or her vision for the organization, had ideas about how fundraising should be conducted. As the young and inexperienced newcomer, I had very little success in completing tasks on time due to the multiple and often conflicting input I received from my colleagues. After my initiation by fire, I learned how to be assertive and diplomatic, which was not an easy task.

THE ART OF COLLABORATION

The most interesting experiences I had in development were a series of meetings with a group of employees from several organizations. In response to current budget constraints and the philanthropic emphasis on collaboration, our organization joined with several others for two different initiatives. The first project aimed to develop a loan fund for child-care providers so they could expand their facilities and resources. The individuals involved in designing the plan for this project included a corporate banker, a marketing specialist, and three executive directors of nonprofit organizations, each very different in mission. I went to my first meeting because our executive director was unable to attend, and I was included for several months thereafter. It was a fortunate occurrence for me, because I learned a great deal about management, presentation, and the complexity of collaborative efforts.

More important than the organizations involved were the individual philosophies and personalities that converged at these meetings. Meetings were held to discuss the fundraising plan for the project, the marketing materials, and the actual design and implementation of the loan fund. At first I was charged with the responsibility of creating a general grant proposal for the project. Financial institutions and foundations were the primary targets. I had not been in my position for very long, and I was thrilled with the idea of playing such a part in the development of the project. Since I was present at the meetings, I was able to participate and share my ideas. I contributed to discussions about training child-care providers and the materials used to recruit borrowers and funders. Without the restrictions of a particular grant application or guidelines, I was exhilarated by this chance to affect the outcome and development of a project, especially since I was in the company of experts who had been working in their respective fields for many years.

This project began with the idea that the three organizations involved—a child-care organization, a facilities development fund, and a law organization—would share the work equally and therefore share the resources equally. Thrown into this mix was a very active marketing consultant and a banking adviser involved in the funding and planning process. As it turned out, the division of labor was skewed based on the specialties of the organizations.

My participation in these meetings was short-lived, and soon I was simply an observer of the dynamics of this collaboration. Eventually it was decided that the marketing consultant would take over the responsibility of fundraising for this project. When they needed me to write proposals for the project, I would be called with very little time left before the deadline, and I had to gather information from each of the parties involved. Usually this meant I would drop my current workload, always bountiful, and dedicate several days to this project. Often the most difficult part of my work was having to incorporate the input of several sources. I was the young writer, not a professional in the legal field, and I was given a multitude of criticisms and suggestions. The problem did not lie in the existence of such feedback but rather the need for other people to control the final product and review it several times. Each individual had his or her agenda for the presentation, depending on his or her background. I encountered a proprietary spirit that I had not anticipated. In the midst of this collaboration, which was quite successful in its fundraising efforts, at least one participant felt neglected at all times. Eventually my supervisor intervened and insisted that each person be given only one chance to review a draft of the proposals. With his authority as manager he was able to take this action, whereas I had been unable to stop that cycle.

The second collaborative project was designed as a one-stop shopping initiative to aid organizations suffering from the drastic changes occurring in the nonprofit environment. The mission statement of this project embodied the goals of the new trends in nonprofit work. An organization would complete a common application and would have access to the resources of all of the participating organizations, including legal counsel, facilities development, fundraising consulting, marketing, and administrative and accounting assistance. In theory this project was ideal, and the initial funding was easy to obtain. However, once again the problem of imbalance had not been anticipated.

At the end of the first year, the organizations had to concede to themselves and the funding agency that it had not been a great success. However, the discussion surrounding this admission was productive. The issue of balance once again became the focus. One of the most important tasks when working in a difficult and changing environment is setting reasonable goals. This team, in its excitement, had signed on to an enormous amount of work that could not be accomplished within the constraints of time and funding. Rather than forging ahead with unreasonable ambition, the group stopped long enough to reevaluate its progress and engage the funder in the process of designing the next phase of the project. I was fortunate to observe the treatment of one of the greatest obstacles facing organizations.

JUGGLING

My experience of college and its related activities was that they occupied as much time as I had, expanding to fill my waking hours. When I embarked upon my postcollegiate life, I believed that the structure of working full time would allow me to divide the remainder of my time between social activity and volunteer work. However, while working for a nonprofit organization in which resources were stretched, I found out quickly that any sort of regular time commitment beyond work was more than I could handle. I worked extra hours, commuted thirty to forty-five minutes each way, and my work and the energy I spent thinking about it expanded as I became more involved. I was left with just enough energy to spend some time with my friends.

The toughest and probably the most important lesson I learned from this experience concerns balance. School had required a very specific sort of juggling that had little to do with life outside of the small campus. I had to manage going to class, doing my course work, working part time, spending time with my friends, and participating in extracurricular activities. However, all of this activity was restricted to four or five city blocks, and none of it determined whether I would have enough money to eat or pay my rent. Once I was working full time, I had the same concerns, as well as significant financial and work-related considerations.

TECHNOLOGY

Though our office was not particularly high-tech, it was necessary to produce and access information quickly to survive. I worked in this organization with eleven to fourteen employees at any given time. Administrative support was stretched beyond its limits, and the executive director played the roles of manager, fundraiser, political liaison, and computer network supervisor. We were fortunate to have realtively up-to-date computers with e-mail access, but in such a small office, any technological snafu causes a meltdown. We had an extremely unreliable fax machine and, until just before my departure, a temperamental photocopier. We did a lot of work with large law firms who could send broadcast facsimiles to hundreds of offices with little effort. Contrast this with the image of me spending a weekend printing, folding, stamping, and sealing 400 letters for our annual individual fundraising appeal.

COPING WITH CHANGE

In my last months with this organization, many structural changes occurred and I was able to observe (and participate in) the process of coping with change. During my tenure at the organization, it had become clear to me whenever change was about to occur. I had not invested decades of work in this organization or the field, so I was somewhat detached from the process. I could see the effects that unfamiliar circumstance had on my coworkers. Many of the attorneys had families and had grown used to a certain lifestyle that they believed to be threatened by change.

Two employees left the organization within a short period of time, and some of the personality conflicts between coworkers reared their heads. Our supervisor, who had been exhausted in every sense of the word for several months, decided to delegate much of the work required to get the organization back on track. A mediator was brought in to address the management issues. Two individuals at the same level who had worked together begrudgingly for many years were told essentially that they needed to learn quickly to coexist peacefully. The fiscal officer was given the additional responsibility of managing office operations. Monthly staff meetings were implemented. All of these were positive and proactive responses to change. However, the fact remained that resources were insufficient and morale was low. Two attorneys out of eight left, one of the two support staff was out with a broken leg, and clients were frustrated because their work was not being done. As I was leaving the organization, another woman left, and the instability continued. Just a few months after my departure, another management position was created to relieve the load of the executive director and to supervise the legal staff.

At the same time the executive director was working with the board of directors to implement two new procedures. The first was a customer satisfaction survey designed for both the nonprofit clients and for the pro bono attorneys who worked with our organization. The second project was to develop a system of employee evaluations and compensation; up to this point, raises or bonuses had been awarded based on budget availability and were calculated purely by percentage. These were positive steps toward a healthy organization, but they were slow moving and relied on the work of independent consultants, most of whom had donated their services.

My education in organizational dynamics did not stop with the higher levels of management. I was struck by how much interpersonal relations affected the work environment. Working conditions were determined by the office climate. As I prepared to leave the organization during this period of uncertainty, nerves were raw and everyone was distracted. In several instances, difficulty stemmed from political and personal differences. In these cases, the executive director intervened with a reminder of the organization's policy on harassment. More common, however, were moments of conflict or misunderstanding resulting from a general weariness. Individuals were overworked and concerned about their positions and the future of the organization. In an office environment filled with uncertainty and unpredictability, no one knew quite what results to expect from these new actions. It is not difficult to understand why workers were irritable and afraid. Productivity was reduced and momentum was lacking.

It did not take long to recognize the challenges of working in this organization. What took extra time and effort was trying to figure out my own methods of coping with these challenges. I saw that some of the people surrounding me were unable to leave their work in the office at the end of the day. Others managed to walk away from the office unencumbered. Several elements were involved in my process of learning to manage the stress. First, I could not let my sense of effectiveness be linked to the efficacy of the organization. I was not responsible for the actions of any other member of the organization. I could only control my own role in the creation of grant proposals, and once I had done my part to the best of my ability, I needed to let go of the rest.

Second, in an environment where feedback and guidance were not given often, I had to develop my own sense of self-evaluation. I would check frequently with the consultant about my progress on a particular project. Once I had established a rhythm to working in the organization, it was much easier to feel good, without external reinforcement, about the work I did.

In terms of time and energy management, it took real effort to truly leave my work behind each evening. Occasionally, I did bring actual work home with me, but more difficult was the intangible baggage of the day's work. I had to make a conscious decision not to worry about or discuss work after hours. I found it difficult to socialize with colleagues because work occupied so much of our conversation. In a culture where people spend approximately eight hours a day working, it is difficult to avoid talking about work. However, I recognized that the only way I would escape this trap was to enjoy my time off while I had it.

Ultimately, I had to accept that some of the larger issues were beyond my control. I learned to be assertive where it was appropriate, and I did meet several times to discuss various issues with the executive director. Beyond that, I knew that management conflicts and limits to resources would continue to affect the office environment, but I could not change them. As I mentioned in this book's introduction, I have learned the importance of being able to advocate for oneself. Recognizing the difference between individual and systemic issues was crucial in helping me learn my limits and work effectively in this environment.

A MODEST VISION

The lessons I learned during my tenure with the organization relate directly to the issues addressed in Chapter 2. In addition to my personal time management and negotiations to balance my work life and personal life, I learned significant lessons about effective organizational behavior.

The importance of effective management was immediately apparent to me. In this realm, the lack of follow-up in our office was problematic. Changes in procedures would be made and employees were expected to comply, but our feedback was not considered. There was a vision behind the work of the organization, but individuals did not take the time to investigate whether it was being executed. Better communication was necessary between the management and the other employees and between the organization and its clients.

Flexibility was a key factor in my work. When I started at this organization, I would become frustrated if I did not receive feedback or necessary information promptly. At some point I realized that I would have to move on with my next task and let others work at their own pace. It was equally important for me to set limits with colleagues who had unrealistic expectations. As with any collaborative or community effort, compromise and understanding were essential. Diversity of opinion and work contributed to the energy and productivity levels of the office.

Though I continue to have a strong interest in nonprofit human services work, I must admit that my idealism has been tempered. In the past, working as a volunteer had allowed me a skewed view of this work. For one thing, as a volunteer I was treated differently and praise certainly was more forthcoming. As I entered the working world with little experience in the nonprofit office, I naively believed that a common purpose or vision would be sufficient to create a functional working team and forgot the protection that college had allowed me. My academic experience was just that: a theoretical approach rather than an applied experience. I believed Margaret Mead's declaration about a small group of individuals making a difference. However, her oft-quoted maxim fails to take into account the external factors discussed in this book. My perspective as a new graduate was quite different from that of my coworkers, most of whom had been practicing community development law for at least ten years.

Recently I was offered an exciting position: I was to design and implement a summer program of arts, recreation, and education for a group of children in a low-income housing development. Finally I was being offered an autonomous position providing direct services. As I asked more questions I learned that I would be responsible for as many as a hundred children and would be working without a budget. My initial excitement faded, and I had to accept my own limits as well as those of this well-intentioned nonprofit organization. Ulitmately, that meant missing an opportunity. As I look forward to working in human services, I will retain some of the political idealism that is rooted deeply in my soul. However, I have modified my expectations to meet the reality of a challenging field.

A DIFFERENT APPROACH

Not long after finishing most of the work on this book, I made a transition in my own working life. This shift gave me the opportunity to apply some of the concepts I researched and discussed while writing these chapters and conducting interviews with young people working in human services. My decision to pursue work in direct services was not coincidental—the process of working on this book reminded me of my original goals and encouraged me to take some risks in order to move closer to these goals.

After leaving my position at the legal nonprofit, I took another position in fundraising, this time with a development consulting firm. This firm is a for-profit organization that serves nonprofit organizations with a wide range of development and organizational services. Though I knew the organization and its employees to be fully dedicated to the work of these nonprofits, I was ambivalent about working in a for-profit organization. However, since I was an hourly employee with no benefits, the decision came down to money and a flexible schedule, both of which would be difficult to guarantee in a nonprofit organization.

In this position I moved from writing grants and appeal letters to doing research on funding prospects for clients. I learned some invaluable skills related to choosing viable funding prospects, the timing of proposals, and making the right connections at foundations. In these respects, I built upon the knowledge and skills gained in my first development position. I worked with a variety of nonprofit organizations, expanding my experience to include groups working in education, the arts, economic development and entrepeneurship, social services, public health, and several organizations working on children's health issues. I enjoyed the challenge of narrowing the immense database of foundation information to a finely tuned list of reasonable prospects that would hopefully result in a pool of money for an organization.

In an earlier chapter we discuss how nonprofit organizations are sometimes forced to operate like for-profit corporations to survive in the competitive climate. Ironically, this particular for-profit organization operated much like the model of nonprofit organizations with which I am familiar. Obviously, any discussion on this level runs the risk of over-simplification, which is not my intention. I do not know how much this environment in the consulting firm is a result of working only with nonprofits, many of which struggle to stay afloat. As with my previous employer, human resources were stretched beyond capacity, and capital resources were certainly made to seem scarce. Almost every employee worked very hard and long hours, carried many clients, and felt under-compensated or under-appreciated at some point. During my year with the organization, staff turnover was extraordinary. To the credit of management, they made real and visible efforts to improve the working environment and made admissions when a wrong fit occurred. Communication was very important in principle but not always in practice. Staff meetings were inconsistent, and informal meetings were difficult to arrange due to busy schedules and varied priorities. Unfortunately, during the times when discussion might have been most useful, stress and preoccupation with the bottom line prevented it. We were told many times how many clients the firm was taking and how much work existed, and everyone acknowledged the hard work and pressure to perform quickly and excellently, but limiting the number of clients was not discussed.

Once again I found myself working in an environment where the work far exceeded the capabilities of the staff, which was at least two people short of capacity. I became frustrated by the situation because I rarely heard when I was doing good work but always heard when we were not meeting expectations. Also, I began to feel that I was doing work that surpassed the compensation I received. The results of my attempts to address these issues were not satisfactory, though I did find my supervisors willing to engage in discussion. While working on this book and evaluating my postcollegiate employment up to this point, I decided that I needed to make a transition from development work, which allowed other people to implement direct service programs, to doing some of that work myself.

INITIATION BY FIRE: MOVING TO DIRECT SERVICES

Ultimately, I decided to leave New York and when I did so, I began to look for work in direct human services. I was in a difficult position because I found myself in a new city starting over. Though I had been out of college for several years, I was pursuing positions for which I had no training. Several people agreed to meet with me for informational interviews and all of them agreed to contact me within a week. Despite my persistence, none of these initial contacts ever followed through with their promises. My desire for instant gratification was squelched. I knew from the start that any position I took would pay much less than my previous position, and I was willing to make this sacrifice. Yet this job search made me feel like I was begging people to let me work for next to nothing. I took a position working in a restaurant until I found something related to my goals. And, after a couple of months, I found a job!

The position I accepted was as a staff member in a group home that serves boys ages ten to twenty-one who are mentally retarded and have various other physical and emotional conditions. The program is run by the subsidiary of a large national managed care organization. Once again, I was faced with the dilemma of working under a for-profit umbrella. I decided that it was an exciting opportunity and the program and atmosphere of the home had been described to me in a way that seemed consistent with my own philosophy. The importance of communication was emphasized and it was made clear that the care of the two residents was the top priority. In short, the concerns of the corporate world seemed distant enough from the day-to-day work of the group home.

My first challenge occurred before I even started working. It took over one month from the time I was informally offered the position to the day that I was able to start working. Part of this delay was due to timing (the end of the calendar year) and procedures necessary to work with children, such as criminal background checks, but much of the delay was a result of corporate bureaucracy. It seemed like every other day I had to fill out more paperwork, pay for another test or obtain a new document proving that I was fit to work in this setting. I do not mean to criticize caution, because I recognize its importance when it concerns the care of children, but I felt like I was spinning my wheels. Once all of these steps were taken and my employment was official, there were many more waivers and documents, and, finally, my training in the home.

I was quite nervous and exhilarated during the first week. My first two days were with the group home supervisor, who explained the day-to-day operations of the home and the company policies. Many of these policies and procedures were determined by the documentation requirements of Medicaid and other outside funding sources. My supervisor touched upon the philosophy of the program during this orientation, but most of the training was very fairly technical in nature. Despite my desire for more information on the conceptual basis of a fairly complex behavioral program, I appreciated the concrete instruction. In the past I had been rushed into working with a strong theoretical introduction to the organization's work but without much technical training.

After these two days of orientation, I began my on-the-job training, the first phase of which involved observing two shifts in the home. This opportunity to familiarize myself with the residents and the operations of the program was a great relief compared to the "sink or swim" approach I had begun to expect. These first days were somewhat awkward. During those initial training shifts some staff members seemed to have no interest in helping or even talking to me. The residents, two teenage boys, were as open to my presence as they would be to a stranger. In fact, I discovered later that they were on their best behavior! It was difficult for me to begin to form my relationships with the residents or staff while I was present only as a peripheral observer.

Much of my early discomfort was reasonable since I was a new employee entering a small and pre-established community. This fact was painfully obvious to me during my first staff meeting, which occurred during my first week. Everyone was welcoming and kind, but the shared experience of the group ran deep and I felt like an outsider. Race was an added factor in my feeling outside of the group. All of the residents and employees of the home are African-American. Nobody made me feel unwelcome because I am white, but it was a fact noticed by all and another way in which I was different from the group.

After these two training shifts, I began to work as a regular employee in the home. Almost immediately challenges presented themselves that I could not have anticipated. One extensive conversation during my initial orientation days concerned the aggressive behavior of one of the residents. This theme was echoed in most of my early interactions with other staff members. Once I began working with this resident, it was clear that what had been emphasized was his behavior and its unpleasant effects rather than suggestions of how to respond to this behavior, or more importantly, the ways in which we might help prevent this behavior. The first several times I worked with this resident I felt quite unprepared and alone. This discomfort resulted in fear, which made me ineffective in working with him. My initial attempts to express my concerns to my colleagues and supervisor were mostly met with responses like "You'll get used to it. It just takes time." Unfortunately, I was not comfortable adopting this attitude. I knew that it was not therapeutic for me or the resident if I viewed him as a threat. He is, after all, a child in my care. One day he began to throw things at me every time I spoke to him. I was petrified and I knew that he could sense my fear, so I became very upset. Fortunately my supervisor was in the house and I was able to communicate to her how uncomfortable I was in the situation. I was frustrated that it took such an extreme reaction to generate productive discussion. After several months, there are still aspects of the work for which I feel unprepared or that make me uncomfortable, but I have made steady progress.

During the time that I have worked at the home, I have worked with almost every staff member and witnessed the incredibly varied styles of the staff. As time passes and I am exposed to these different approaches, I am able to find my own comfort level and style of working within the program. I have discovered that the diversity of methods presents some major complications. Since the program is rooted in behavior modification and the use of goal sheets and concrete results, consistency is crucial to its success. I have found that the differences in staff approaches go far beyond personality types. Some staff do not adhere to the policies or even the philosophy of the program. When working in the midst of challenging or unpleasant behavior, it is natural to try approaches that will stop this behavior. However, I see some staff members doing anything to make the negative aspects of the work go away, such as appeasing the resident by giving him what he wants even when policy dictates otherwise or putting him to bed when he becomes uncooperative. These inconsistencies are not fair to other staff members, but more importantly, they damage our shared mission, which is to care for the residents. Enabling negative behavior does not encourage change.

While communication of all kinds is encouraged in theory, I have not found it to be welcomed in practice at all times. When I began working in the home, my supervisor showed me the staff communication book, which I thought was a brilliant idea. Since no more than two staff members are ever in the house at one time, this book gives staff an opportunity to pass along any information to everyone else in a structured way. In reality, this book is used almost exclusively by the supervisors to reprimand staff for errors in documentation or unfulfilled duties. Similarly, staff meetings, as in previous settings, are often used as a forum for complaints. To her credit, my supervisor did plan one meeting entirely dedicated to boosting morale and socializing over dessert. I was impressed by her awareness of the difficulty of working in this environment and her effort to re-energize staff. I rarely find the content of the meetings or the written comments offensive or unfounded, but the tone in which they are presented seems condescending or accusatory. Individuals tend to get so caught up in making their own needs clear that they ignore the interactive quality of communication. Especially when tension is high, I find it crucial to be aware how language is received by other people.

While my experience in this position is dramatically different from my fundraising positions, it has reinforced many of the lessons I learned in those situations, as well as the themes discussed throughout this book. All of the forces that influence organizations and promote or hinder change, are evident in this program. The largest force present in all these situations is economics. Much of our program is determined by corporate policies or the reporting requirements of outside agencies that control the finances of the program. Many of the policies of these agencies are shaped by federal and state politics and legislation, especially when it comes to subsidized care for these children. As illustrated by my earlier examples, interpersonal dynamics and larger social forces have a significant impact on the work we do and the overall effectiveness of the program. The purchase of equipment medically necessary for one of the residents was delayed by three weeks because my supervisor had to wait for the approval of the Department of Social Services. Even technology plays a larger role than one might expect. While we do not rely on computers to provide direct services, we do rely on telephones as access to the outside world, and the group home's telephone lines have mysteriously stopped working several times during my brief tenure. While the clients are supposed to be the most important elements of the program, their needs often seem subservient to these larger forces.

CHANGING PERSPECTIVE

Currently I work in another position providing direct services. I am a long-term temporary teacher in a school within a psychiatric hospital. I work mostly with elementary school children. My day is split between working with children who are hospitalized short term for crisis stabilization who are in school only a couple of hours per day and the long term residential- or day-treatment students, who attend school all day. The student body has a lot in common with the population of the group home, though most of the students are not as severely developmentally delayed. Though I cannot address many of the larger forces at work within the organization, since I am a new and temporary member of this team, it is clear to me that all of the same forces do influence the operations of the school. Besides the obvious differences and the fact that the school is a public program, the primary difference between my experiences in these two settings is the amount of actual reliable support I receive on a daily basis. In the group home the only adults present, no matter what the situation, are the two staff members on duty, each one assigned to one resident. We can call our supervisor or even the police if we require outside intervention, but our immediate resources are limited. In the school there are other teachers present who are willing to help each other, as well as extremely competent hospital staff. Not only does this mean that I feel much more a part of a team, but the students have access to much more support, especially when making choices about their behavior. Their teachers, peers, therapists and unit staff are all within reach throughout the day. I have found this setting to be more compatible with my personal style and needs. This revelation, however, presents a dilemma. Philosophically, I am much more inclined to work in small, community-based programs. I am not interested in negotiating the many complications of a large bureaucratic infrastructure. Nevertheless, I have experienced the tangible benefits of a large, well-staffed facility.

For me the shift from consulting to direct services has been gratifying. What has surprised me in my current work are not the differences between working in direct human services and working in development but the shared traits in all of the experiences. The greatest difference between my current and previous experiences is how I feel about doing the work. I am no less frustrated by the obstacles or injustices I encounter. However, I feel much more fulfilled by the work I do each day. I love working with children and not sitting at a computer typing all day. I still believe that my previous work was valuable, but now I feel that I am contributing to the lives of people I see every day. The results of my work are tangible though not always immediately apparent. I would not be honest if I did not admit to the selfish aspects of the work. The best part of making a change in my professional life is the reward I reap from this work—the satisfaction I feel when I finish my day, a feeling that can even overpower the physical exhaustion of having worked a very long and difficult shift.

One of the questions I discussed with other young people working in human services concerned our preparation for this work. Many of them addressed formal and informal aspects of their undergraduate experiences that did or did not prepare them for their postcollegiate work. For the most part, these individuals did not feel well-equipped with the necessary tools. I would have to echo this sentiment emphatically, with one exception. My studies, even in women's studies and the social sciences, did not and could not prepare me for the actual experience of providing direct services.

The exception I would make to this sense of being unprepared concerns the concept of community. My undergraduate experience, both academic and social, taught me a great deal about the importance of community and of communication within community. I became frustrated at times with the emphasis on process rather than progress within the college. Now I treasure the lessons I learned working closely with others to resolve conflicts or create solutions within academic classes, college organizations and residence halls. My experience in human services thus far has demonstrated the importance of community repeatedly. Although there have been many similarities in the various settings, the sense of cohesiveness or fragmentation has varied significantly. The ease/unease of communication, the willingness/refusal of individuals to help each other, and the investment/apathy toward building a sense of collaboration or community have had major effects on the way in which I am able to deal with obstacles and do my job effectively. The ways in which individual members of organizations treat each other and the models presented to encourage/discourage community-building have proven to be much more important to me than the details of the setting or the size of the organization.

POINTS TO PONDER

1. Have you done volunteer work in human services? Have you been employed full-time in human services? How have these experiences differed?

2. At this point, what would your ideal position be? Can you imagine some of the challenges you would face in this situation?

3. Are young people who have grown up in an environment of rapid change better able to cope with the current human services environment? If so, in what ways are they better prepared?

4. Identify several links between the narrative of this chapter and the trends described in Chapter 2. Do you see a connection between the theories or organizations and the events described by the author?

Designing Change: Organizational Perspectives

Applying the Concepts of Change

- You are the newest employee of a small nonprofit health clinic. Your first
  project is to redesign the brochures that will be sent into the community
  to advertise for services. Our supervisor asks you to finish your draft and
  circulate it to the office so "everyone can take a look." When you check
  your mailbox on Monday morning, it is full of lengthy critiques of and
  suggestions for the brochure. You know that tension is high this week
  after employee evaluations, and there are politics under the surface that
  you do not understand yet. Your supervisor has asked you to finish the
  brochure and send it to the printer by Tuesday morning. You have two
  meetings and a long list of people to call on Monday. How would you
  approach the situation? If you decide to discuss the issue with your
  supervisor, what are your reservations?

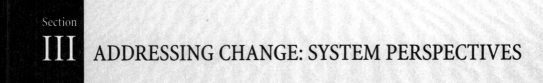

Section

III ADDRESSING CHANGE: SYSTEM PERSPECTIVES

CHAPTER 7

INTO THE LION'S DEN
Understanding the Dynamics of a Large State Agency

Many organizations are not run in such a way as to recognize that the welfare of individuals is at stake.

— Matthew P. Dumont, M.D., Psychiatrist

M ost people have strong views on how central government agencies impact the lives of citizens. Less is known about the actual internal dynamics of these organizations. In this chapter we get a glimpse of the inner workings of a large state mental health agency. Examples of why and how policies are established and decisions are made are presented within the framework of political, economic, social, and programmatic forces described in Chapter 1. In addition to examining how the agency operates, attention is also given to what it is like to work in a complex, bureaucratic organization and how staff cope with the frustrations that exist at this level of government.

While most change-oriented individuals begin with the assumption that one's intervention will have a significant impact on the target system, it took only a modest degree of reality testing to reach the conclusion that such a goal was not possible in this situation. This chapter also describes the goals and activities of the agency, the environmental dynamics of the work setting, the responses of those who work in that environment, and the ways in which one individual attempted to apply an organizational/systems development perspective to this setting.

~

Before working in the New York State Office of Mental Health I had spent most of my professional career in small- or medium-size work settings. I knew that it would be different working in a large system, but I was not fully prepared for the magnitude of the operation and the impact it has on those who work in it. While it is difficult to convey a comprehensive picture of this system in a brief chapter, perhaps a few facts and figures will illustrate the enormous size and scope of this system.

The New York State Office of Mental Health is the largest mental health agency in the world. Until 1978, the Office of Mental Health was a division of the Department of Mental Hygiene, which encompassed divisions for mental retardation and developmental disabilities; alcoholism; and mental health. After becoming an independent agency, the Office of Mental Health had a budget of more than $975 million of state funding in 1981. When other sources of funding, such as Medicaid, are included, the total amount of money spent in the public mental health system in New York State was $1.5 billion.

In 1980, 39,000 people were employed directly by the State Office of Mental Health. That number did not include county personnel or staff of provider agencies under contract to the state.

Also at that time, approximately 25,000 inpatients were in state-operated facilities, a dramatic reduction from the 93,000 inpatients in 1955 and 78,000 in 1968. Considering that there were only approximately 140,000 residents of mental hospitals in the entire country, New York State had more than 15 percent of the total psychiatric inpatients in the United States.

In addition to persons served by state inpatient facilities, over 500,000 people received mental health services in the public mental health system in 1980. These individuals were served by a series of mental health systems, including state, county, and municipal programs, as well as community mental health centers, general hospitals, and other voluntary agencies providing mental health services. In any geographic area, many or all of these provider types may be operating under a variety of governance auspices, usually in a fragmented and uncoordinated manner. In many instances, the planning, reporting, budgeting, and personnel mechanisms are different for each system, creating a myriad of problems for delivering effective, comprehensive services in an integrated manner.

Most often clients are forced to follow the funding sources, rather than the more desirable alternative of dollars following clients. It is not difficult to understand this dynamic when one considers that a single agency may have at least twelve sources of funding for its program. Of the federal funding sources, only 12.5 percent come from mental health agencies. The remaining 87.5 percent come from other sources, such as social services and vocational rehabilitation.

How does someone accustomed to working in a small community-based setting approach this mind-boggling situation? How does one understand the dynamics of a large, intricate system and then apply this knowledge to changing complex, multiprogram service delivery systems? These are the questions I pondered as I began working for the New York State Office of Mental Health. It did not take long for me to realize that I had omitted a very critical question from my consideration. It was not enough to think about how to deal with the system; it also was necessary to give serious attention to the question of how I would cope with the system and how I would survive, at least in the psychological sense.

ADJUSTING TO A NEW ENVIRONMENT

Having never worked in the central office of a large government organization, I had only my stereotypes to rely on as I tried to anticipate this experience. The popular view of a bureaucratic headquarters was of a place where nothing happened, nobody cared, and everyone counted the days until retirement. While I would not go so far as to describe the workplace I entered as idyllic, certainly these stereotypes did not apply. I found a fast-paced environment, inhabited by people with a great deal of energy and visions of system change guiding their activities. Of course, my position as associate commissioner of program development placed me within the executive management level of the agency. However, the contact I had with workers at all levels confirmed my impression that the bureaucracy was neither heartless nor mindless. This is not to suggest that self-actualization and community spirit prevailed. There certainly were problems. However, it was not until later that I was able to appreciate how these behaviors, which seemed so incongruous to me, were actually coping mechanisms and self-preservation responses.

MAJOR GOALS AND DIRECTIONS OF THE AGENCY

I joined the central office staff in 1978. The deinstitutionalization movement, with its emphasis on shifting individuals with mental disabilities from institutions to community settings, had been completed. In New York State, the number of individuals residing in state psychiatric centers was less than one-third of what it had been ten years earlier. Thousands of mentally disabled individuals populated urban centers and smaller communities contiguous to state psychiatric facilities. Many of these individuals had inadequate housing and virtually no employment or recreational opportunities. In addition, their lack of coping and social skills and their unusual appearance made it difficult for them to participate as members of the communities in which they lived. The situation was made even worse by the hostility and resistance of the established members of these communities.

The growing concern about the presence and plight of the mentally disabled who moved from institution to community brought to the forefront an awareness that simply moving people from institutions to community settings was not enough. Advocates, providers, and policy makers, as well as other concerned citizens, realized that the basic supports provided within institutions—shelter, food, a sense of security—had not been taken into account under the policy of deinstitutionalization. As destructive as institutions were, they did provide sustenance and asylum in the positive sense.

If individuals with chronic mental disabilities and long histories of institutional dependence were to survive and function effectively in community settings, it would be necessary to provide a viable system of services and supports.

At the same time, it was recognized that in spite of the rapid decline of institutions during the past decade, it was unrealistic to expect that inpatient psychiatric facilities would disappear, at least within the foreseeable future. The large numbers of frail elderly individuals who had resided in these institutions for decades, and the need for a protective environment for those whose mental impairments made them dangerous to self or others, ensured the continued existence of these facilities.

In response to these psychiatric, sociological and political forces, the Office of Mental Health had set an overall goal of establishing a comprehensive and coordinated system of mental health services in each geographic area. In order to achieve this goal and concurrently redistribute resources from institutional to community settings, the office established two major interim initiatives:

- Movement toward community-based services through the development of community support systems providing a full range of mental health and life support services and opportunities.

- Improvement of the quality of care within psychiatric facilities.

VEHICLES FOR ACHIEVING GOALS

The first step in implementing this mission was the development of a comprehensive conceptual framework. After considering several conceptual frameworks, including the Community Support System and the Balanced Service Systems models, the office settled on a hybrid version that provided a continuum of service along the major life support dimensions. Not only did this enable the office to describe all of the key elements of the service system, but it also provided a common set of descriptive terms and definitions to be used for planning, budgeting, management, monitoring, and evaluation. Given the fragmented, confusing patterns of service delivery, it was considered essential to have a common service template. This template had to be comprehensive enough to take into account all important service elements and broad enough to allow for individual differences within the diverse array of geographic settings within the state.

Having established a common framework, a number of other system change mechanisms were established. These included the following:

• *Reduction of the inpatient census by 5,000 individuals within the next five years.* Since more than 80 percent of the state mental health budget was allocated to inpatient settings and it was unlikely that more total resources would be given to the mental health system, it became necessary to reduce the size of the inpatient system in order to make resources available for the development of a community-based system. The only viable ways to achieve this shift would be to reduce the number of inpatient residents, thus freeing staff to be moved to community settings and close psychiatric facilities in order to reduce enormous maintenance costs. While political factors made it difficult to close a psychiatric center—not a single state-operated psychiatric center had ever been closed in New York State despite the 75 percent census reduction—the office decided to develop a proposal for consolidating and closing several facilities.

• *Enhancement of service integration through the development of case management, core service agencies, and management districts.* Fragmentation and lack of continuity were serious and pervasive problems at all levels, from providing direct service to clients to coordinating the efforts of the multiple agencies and levels of government responsible for meeting the mental health needs of the state's citizens. The existence of a large state system and a strong voluntary agency and county government presence—often functioning in a parallel and unrelated manner—produced discontinuity and duplication of effort that impeded the delivery of comprehensive and holistically oriented services and led to inefficient and wasteful use of resources.

• *Development of rational and coordinated funding mechanisms necessary to counteract the negative influence of current ways in which services were paid for.* While almost everyone agreed that current funding practices served as a disincentive to delivering services in a manner that met the needs of individuals seeking help, service providers were reluctant to accept a system that would threaten their ability to balance the books by imposing eligibility requirements and other forms of accountability. On the other hand, funding sources, fearful of losing control, resisted proposals that combined funding streams in order to facilitate needs-based planning and service delivery. Despite several futile attempts to promote a unified funding mechanism, the office continued to explore funding approaches that would support effective and efficient delivery of services based on individual needs.

• *Active pursuit of a policy of maximizing the use of mainstream services to deliver human services to the mentally disabled.*   The previous emphasis on removal from the community and total institutional care had reinforced the sense of segregation and isolation experienced by the persons with chronic mental disabilities and had increased the stigma associated with mental health problems. In order to reverse this pattern and affirm the disabled individual's right to equal treatment within the community, the office worked with other state-level human services agencies to ensure access to the same social, health, recreational, employment, and educational services as other members of the community.

A Framework for Observing and Analyzing This Setting

Being a psychologist with a community perspective, I naturally attempted to make sense of my experience in state government using the conceptual tools that were most familiar to me. While I was initially overwhelmed by the size, pace, complexity, and unfamiliar administrative language, after a while I began to understand how the system operated.

   A large central government agency, like any other organization, can be understood in political, psychological, sociological, cultural, and economic terms. In my analysis of this complex organizational structure, I relied on a variety of theoretical approaches, including social systems and dynamic and behavioral paradigms. I found that although it was not possible to gain a full understanding of the setting with any single conceptual model, valuable insights could be gained from each perspective. For example, while the political influences within this setting are pervasive, it is necessary to employ concepts derived from individual psychology to understand how individuals at each level of the hierarchy respond to these forces. In the same manner, one cannot fully comprehend individual behavior patterns without taking into account the ecological structure of the system. (See the following sections for specific illustrations).

Before describing the details of this experience, let me offer one of the basic conclusions I reached:

> *State government as a community setting is not qualitatively different from other settings; the differences are primarily quantitative.*

FACTORS AND FORCES INFLUENCING BEHAVIOR IN THIS SETTING

What are the major variables affecting behavior in the public mental health system? Certainly the factors and theories of psychology and psychiatry provide a conceptual base for planning and implementing services. Likewise, the philosophical and ethical principles underlying the concern for individual rights and human welfare set a standard for people working in this setting. However, my experience in the central office underscored the prominent influence of other sources of influence—factors that I knew existed but whose impact I had not truly appreciated.

Consider the following examples of how forces that are not primarily programmatic affect the ways in which the New York State mental health system serves the mentally disabled:

Money   One of the most serious obstacles to serving persons with chronic mental disabilities in community settings is the lack of access to facilities that provide physical health care. Many long-term residents of state psychiatric centers have only minor psychiatric problems but are suffering from debilitating physical health conditions. Particularly among the elderly, the major impediment to community placement is inadequate access to skilled nursing and health-related facilities.

At first blush, lack of access appears to stem from the fear and resistance of health-care providers regarding the mentally disabled. However, on closer examination, a number of other significant obstacles become apparent. While social attitudes certainly play a role, the financial disincentives associated with the local Medicaid share requirement and the absence of local contribution to maintenance of individuals in state psychiatric centers in New York State serve as even more serious barriers to access.

For example, the cost of maintaining an individual in a New York State psychiatric center in 1981 was approximately $125 per day. This was paid completely by state funding, with some reimbursement from federal Medicaid.

On the other hand, because of the scarcity of nursing-home beds, backlogs of individuals who occupy beds in acute hospital settings at a cost of $300 to $400 per day were ready for health facility placement. Taking space that may be needed by persons with acute medical problems, these individuals often cost local departments of social services $75 to $100 per day in required local Medicaid contributions. If such individuals in the state psychiatric center had been moved into nursing homes, local government would have had to begin paying a 25 percent local Medicaid share. Thus, keeping these individuals in the state psychiatric center allowed the local government to save money, while people in acute hospitals who were competing for the same beds constituted a financial burden for the counties.

Is it any surprise, then, that the chronically mentally disabled have difficulty moving from inappropriate placement in state psychiatric centers to local health-related facilities?

The sheltered workshop provides another example of how funding mechanisms adversely influence service delivery. Sheltered workshops are divided into a series of program activity areas, organized according to the functional capabilities of the clients. As an individual becomes more competent, he or she moves up to a higher-level program activity.

Unfortunately, financial support for these program areas often comes from a variety of unrelated funding sources. The separate funding streams not only create problems of program management and accountability but, in some instances, also provide disincentives for appropriate service delivery. For example, if a person participated in a day treatment program targeted at persons functioning at a fairly low level, the sheltered workshop was reimbursed at a rate of $32 per day. When the individual progressed to the point where he or she could enter a more advanced sheltered work program, the provider was confronted with the dilemma of wanting to provide an opportunity for higher-level functioning for the individual but also being aware that this promotion would lead to a loss of revenue since the higher-level sheltered work program was reimbursed at a rate of less than $9.50 per day.

In an era when operating expenses were rising and funds were becoming more difficult to obtain, this fiscal disincentive served as an additional obstacle to rational treatment and service planning.

Politics   A seasoned veteran of state government once told me that policy decisions are influenced by three factors, in ascending order of influence: human need, fiscal benefit, and political impact. My experience in state government did little to challenge the validity of this line of reasoning.

The influence of political forces was not limited to major policy issues; day-to-day operations also were affected significantly. For instance, the commissioner of the agency was an exceptionally intelligent and competent clinician and administrator. He was a man whose abilities were well-suited for the complex policy and program issues confronting the head of a large state agency. Yet, I rarely sat through a meeting in his office without having him interrupted by a phone call from a legislator or a legislative staff member asking him to ensure rapid admission to the local psychiatric facility for someone's mother-in-law or next-door neighbor. The task of administering this enormous agency was certainly difficult enough without the constant intrusions that should have been appropriately handled at a different level, but could not be ignored by him for fear of future reprisal.

The following examples represent some of the ways in which political forces influence behavior in this setting.

• In 1978, the office embarked upon a major program to provide community support services to individuals with chronic mental disabilities living in community settings. This program, which was a planned response to the problems of deinstitutionalization, was designed not only to provide supports and services in community settings but also to encourage local ownership of community services. In order to achieve this purpose, the office decided to direct all funds from this program to local government and voluntary agencies. However, this intention was not to be fulfilled.

The state employees' union, fearing that the community support effort would eventually lead to a reduction in the state workforce, took full advantage of the fact that it was a gubernatorial election year. The union mounted a strong media campaign accusing the state of "dumping" psychiatric patients into unprepared and overcrowded communities. An intense negotiation ensued, resulting in the issuance of a policy memorandum from the governor's office. The memorandum directed the Office of Mental Health to allocate 50 percent of the community support funds to programs operated by state psychiatric centers. In addition, the agency was told to establish a retraining program that would eventually prepare 6,000 state psychiatric hospital employees to work in community settings.

While it is certainly reasonable to argue that state employees have interests and experience that would be useful in serving the mentally disabled in community settings, this policy directive represented a reversal of the initial decision to reinforce local commitment and responsibility for community-based services. On the other hand, the negotiation yielded two other byproducts: The union did not oppose the governor in his bid for election, and a new media campaign was initiated by the union describing the humane and effective efforts the state was making to serve the mentally disabled in community settings.

• One afternoon, while I was chairing an interagency task force meeting, my secretary whispered to me that I was to report immediately to the commissioner's conference room for an urgent meeting. Upon arriving in the room I was told that a private hospital in a politically sensitive area of the state had been forced to close. The governor, wanting to be responsive to the constituents and legislators of that district, had promised to fund an alternative program, using some of the facility and retaining a portion of the workforce. He instructed large agencies to contribute $250,000 and small agencies to set aside $100,000 during the coming year for this program. The precise purpose and nature of the program were not yet determined; that was why the meeting had been called.

Staff were given four hours to design a multipurpose program that would be responsive to the needs of residents of the affected area. By coincidence, I had recently designed a service program in response to a study conducted in another part of the state. This proposed program, which had not received funding for its original purpose, appeared to be compatible with the expressed needs of the community in which the hospital was being closed. Therefore, this program design was accepted and a large amount of money was committed to the project. Ironically, similar program needs had been articulated in other areas of the state for several years, but efforts to secure funding had been futile.

• If the proverbial Martian were to tour the mental health system of any of the local communities in New York State, the first question she would ask is "Who's in charge?" In any sizeable community there may be dozens of agencies providing mental health services. These agencies operate under a variety of auspices, including state and local government, voluntary and proprietary organizations, individual practitioners, and even the federal government, as in the case of the Veterans Administration. While some channels of responsibility and accountability exist, there is a good deal of uncertainty and ambiguity about how the service system is coordinated and managed. Authority is vested in several agencies—particularly county departments of mental health and the state office of mental health. However, in the absence of a single clearly defined governance structure we find fragmentation and duplication of services, as well as continual bickering about who should be making planning, management, and service delivery decisions.

The cumulative effect of this governance dilemma is a confusing and sometimes chaotic service delivery system whose major players spend a lot of time and energy attempting to clarify issues of authority and responsibility. This situation frustrates and demoralizes direct service delivery personnel, and, of course, the most serious negative consequences are experienced by those individuals with disabilities who are at the receiving end of the service delivery system. These individuals' interests often become lost in the heat of these territorial battles.

Our Martian visitor might wonder why such an obvious problem hasn't been resolved by the educated and knowledgeable people in this field. Although there is no simple answer to this question, a number of factors appear to be contributing to the governance problem. First, since control of fiscal resources is a major source of power, and there are multiple funding sources in this system, it is natural that authority conflicts arise among the various funding auspices, particularly local and state government. Second, historically, local and state government have played very different roles in the delivery of mental health services. Traditionally, state government, through its psychiatric institutions, has assumed responsibility for very disturbed, chronically mentally disabled individuals whose families have not had financial resources to provide private care. On the other hand, local government has tended to serve people living in the community whose disabilities have not been as severe or chronic. As the prevailing philosophy shifted from an institutional base to a community-based approach for serving those with chronic disabilities, these traditional roles no longer applied. The shift to community-based services has resulted in considerable role diffusion and uncertainty, making it difficult to define clearly who is responsible for various target populations.

The final suggested source of the governance dilemma is the political and legal structure of the state. A careful reading of the New York State mental hygiene laws reveals a great deal of ambiguity in relation to the issue of who is in charge. One section of the law designates the state commissioner as having responsibility for planning, coordination, and management services. In another section of the law, these functions are ascribed to the county mental health directors. It is difficult to believe that the assignment of dual responsibility, without clarification of the relationship between the two governing bodies, is accidental. Given the existence of both strong county government and a strong state-operated system, including a powerful state employees union, it is quite possible that the ambiguous legal description of the governance process represents the legislature's attempt to mollify the proponents of both local government and state agency control.

Regardless of the interpretation one places on the mental hygiene laws, it is clear that the political structures' response to the governance issue has made resolution difficult and, without an unequivocal governance structure, mental health clients are confronted with an uncoordinated and discontinuous array of services.

In some instances, both fiscal and political forces interact with each other to exert significant influence on behavior and programs in the mental health system. Some examples of how politics and money work in combination include the following:

• In New York State, the number of individuals residing in state psychiatric inpatient facilities had declined approximately 75 percent in twenty-five years. Yet, with this dramatic reduction in census and a strong commitment to redistribute resources to community services, not a single state psychiatric center had been closed in New York State. This puzzling lack of facility reduction was due primarily to the perceived economic impact upon the local community of a facility closing and the legislature's response to this potential problem. Any legislator who was unable to prevent a facility from closing would virtually be ensured of defeat by constituents concerned about loss of jobs and other negative economic consequences. Since there were more than twenty-five state psychiatric centers spread throughout the state, a large number of legislators were affected by this issue. Feeling empathic toward legislators with facilities at risk in their districts, and fearful of this issue arising in their own backyards, legislators had entered an unwritten pact to stand together against the closing of any state psychiatric facility. Meanwhile, 80 percent of the state mental health budget continues to be allocated to an inpatient system serving only a small proportion of individuals experiencing severe mental health problems.

• Perhaps the most serious obstacle to developing adequate community support systems for individuals with chronic mental disabilities is inadequate and inaccessible housing. In New York City, where the general housing stock is limited and living quarters are very expensive, this is a particularly serious problem. However, these preexisting barriers have been further supplemented by events related to social attitudes toward the mentally disabled and other socially disadvantaged groups. For example, one of the major sources of housing for people who have been discharged from state psychiatric facilities are single-room-occupancy apartments and private proprietary housing units. While these facilities are far from idyllic, in many instances they are the only available sources of housing.

In the late 1970s, landlords took advantage of a New York City tax abatement ordinance that provided considerable financial incentive for the owners of single-room-occupancy buildings to convert those dwellings to cooperative apartments for upper-income residents. This ordinance, which provided a twenty-year tax break for owners of converted buildings, was viewed by many as a less-than-subtle attempt to remove from Manhattan the mentally disabled and other socially disadvantaged. From this perspective, the tax abatement ordinance may be seen as a dual expression of New York City's public policy; it encouraged well-to-do citizens to live in Manhattan and informed the socially disadvantaged that they were not welcome. As such, the tax abatement policy was in direct conflict with another public policy, the development of an adequate system of community support for individuals who had historically been relegated to large psychiatric institutions.

Other Influences   In addition to money and politics, a number of other factors and forces shaped behavior—individual and collective—within the setting of a large state government agency. The following were among the major influences:

• *Value conflicts:* Working within this setting magnified many of the basic philosophical issues related to human services. The combined features of having a broad impact yet not being directly in touch with the people being served added a unique dimension to one's philosophical deliberations. For example, the political pressures of that period were primarily directed toward increased protection of the community and, therefore, an orientation of social control. This approach was in conflict with many of the fundamental human services goals of individual growth and self-determination. Maintaining an orientation of client agentry, with all of the social and political demands placed upon the mental health system, was no easy chore.

• *Pace and volume of activity:*   Aside from any of the economic, political, or social forces, the sheer number and speed of events exerted considerable influence on the behavioral dynamics of the agency. The crisis orientation of mental health, exacerbated by its politicization within state government, fostered a frenetic pace, characterized by a strong demand for quick decisions based on data that were generally inadequate. Further compounding this situation was the understandable, but unrealistic, attitude of many central government offices that both change and control of the system could be managed directly by a centralized staff. Trying to do everything, particularly with relatively limited personnel resources, created extreme frustration and confusion. For example, in New York State the mental health agency not only set policy and regulated mental health services but also directly operated a large system of mental health services. Not only was this a Herculean task, but it also created an inherent conflict since there were also local government and voluntary agencies, often serving the same population and competing for mental health funds, which were overseen by the same agency that had direct operational responsibility for the state service system.

Given the stress and frustration of this environment, it is not surprising that the agency frequently reorganized and realigned itself in order to respond more effectively. Unfortunately, organizational change often became a reflex action, a strategy designed with the express intent of improving functioning, but, in fact, actually serving as a temporary diversion from the enormous problems inherent in managing such an unwieldy system. Thus, the activity of reorganizing became functionally autonomous, developing a life cycle of its own.

• *Problems of size and distance:*   Related to the difficulties of working in an environment of perpetual crisis were the problems of managing a complex system with operations spread across a large geographic area. New York State, with its multiplicity of providers and diverse geography and demography, presented unique management challenges, particularly since there were not commonly accepted mechanisms for making this complex system function in a rational manner. Consider the problem of communicating information. Whether the issue was developing a database using information from local service providers or communicating policy from central office to the field, complications always seemed to arise. Like the child's game "Telephone," something was inevitably lost in transmitting information from one point to another.

The dilemma of a multilayered system is that interventions directed at one problem may, in the process, create additional difficulties. For example, in the New York State mental health system, regional offices were introduced to increase the amount of direct contact between agency management staff and service providers. While regional offices succeeded in reducing the span of direct control, the additional layer of the regional office impeded accurate communication of policies and procedures.

• *Basic psychology of communication and problem solving:*   Not all of my experiences in the state agency setting were negative. Occasionally, the introduction of basic group facilitation strategy served to counterbalance the internal complexities and external pressures that were diverting the agency from its primary mission of serving individuals with disabilities. For instance, a number of individuals involved in an interagency task force that I chaired responded quite positively to the experience of information sharing and group problem solving. Their favorable reaction to a relatively simple process reinforced my belief that at least some of the alienation and distress experienced by those who work in a central government setting could be attributed to the lack of attention given to basic communication enhancement and community building processes.

MAKING SENSE OF THE EXPERIENCE

For a moment, let us consider the community support system—one of the major program initiatives of the state mental health authority—as an analogy that may be useful in explaining the dynamics of this setting. The community support system is based upon several guiding principles:

1. Enabling individuals to achieve and feel a sense of competence.
2. Providing social support.
3. Fostering a sense of personal and community identity.

Just as all three of these concepts are important in assisting individuals with handicapping conditions to adapt to community living, they are also relevant to the experience of individual workers in a central government office. Ironically, our inability to pay attention to or put into practice these same principles we promote for others contributes to the inefficiency, lack of personal accountability, and sense of futility we associate with bureaucracy. Granted, politics and economics were the guiding forces that moved the public mental health system away from its stated goals of human services; however, these psychological and sociological factors should also be taken into account.

Most individuals entering state service share the same goals and aspirations as workers in other settings. In addition to wanting to earn a decent living and achieve career mobility and security, these individuals wish to maintain a positive sense of themselves by performing competently and producing measurable achievements. The problem is that the dynamics of the central office setting make it difficult to attain these personal objectives. The political, economic, and ecological forces described above mitigated against competent performance and positive self-esteem. What occurred may be viewed as an organizational domino effect. Those in top leadership positions within the agency were subject to various political demands and pressures. In order to minimize the threat this posed to themselves, they, in turn, delegated these problems to workers at the next level of organizational hierarchy. This delegation continued to proceed rapidly down through the layers of the organization until it landed on the desk of someone who was unable to delegate further. I am not suggesting that delegation is an inappropriate management strategy. The problem is that this passing of work often occurred solely for the purpose of expediency, without taking into account contextual variables such as current work assignments, appropriate problem-solving procedures, and amount of time needed to do jobs properly.

As a result, almost everyone in the organization was aware of not being able to perform competently. People adapted to this loss of competence, sense of threat, and diminished self-esteem by defending themselves. They pulled inward, set up barriers, and developed work patterns that limited the scope of their responsibility in order to avoid additional failures. Before long, the classical symptoms of the bureaucratic stereotype appeared. Doing only what is expected, disregarding work schedules and deadlines other than those most recently dictated by supervisors, and disassociating oneself from having responsibility or being accountable for anything other than a small segment of work contained in one's job description are all indicators that may be attributed to adaptive behavior in a threatening environment. People working in these agencies were not basically uncaring and apathetic. In fact, outside of the work setting they were often concerned and energetic. Instead, their behavior in the workplace may be viewed as an adaptive response to a situation in which they felt a sense of helplessness and an inability to behave in a competent manner. Another sure sign of this syndrome is the serious loss of imagination that pervades this type of work setting.

Incidentally, there is one other reason for applying the support system model to the central office mental health work setting. In addition to the price we pay for not meeting the needs of our own personnel, the failure to see the relevance to our own situation of the guiding principles of the current approach to mental health delivery reinforces the schism between individuals who are "normal" and those who are "mentally disabled" individuals. By refusing to acknowledge that mental health personnel have the same needs for competence and support as those they serve, we are setting up another distinction between "us" and "them."

LESSONS LEARNED

Early in this chapter I referred to the personal impact of this experience as a participant in central government. I learned about administration and finance, I gained a healthy respect for the complexities of the public mental health system, and I learned a great deal about the politics of state government. However, the most significant lesson that I and others who entered this system with me learned was less intellectual and more personal.

One day, while returning from a particularly frustrating meeting, I began ruminating about my experience at the central office. I considered my usual litany of rationalization: The agency is too expedient; we should resist political pressures; if only I were in charge; I should be back in the field working with real problems.

Finally, having exhausted my usual supply of ruminations, a new idea entered my consciousness. I realized that I was projecting most of my frustration onto external sources: the agency, the system, the field of mental health. While these were certainly genuine sources of concern, there was a more personal basis for my tension. What really mattered were the things I was learning about myself as I worked in this complex and stressful setting. The pace and pressures of the system were forcing me to confront my own behavior and the extent to which it was consistent—or inconsistent—with my perceived values and self-image. As a result, I realized that working in a central government agency was actually an exercise in values clarification.

And what were these value issues? Basically, the self-confrontation revolved around the conflict between being productive and meeting the demands of the work situation, on the one hand, and maintaining a personal and interpersonal style of behavior consistent with one's self-image, both as a professional and an individual. Following are some of the major concerns I observed, both in myself and in others:

- Conflict between an interpersonal-humanistic orientation and a mechanical approach endemic to a bureaucratic, product-oriented work environment.
- Awareness of delusions of grandeur stemming from the belief that working in the central office will enable one to change the system.
- Tension resulting from attempting to create a balance between producing a product and maintaining a constructive problem-solving and work process.
- Conflict between the heavy demands at work and adequate attention to family.
- Ensuring survival of the "self" within an impersonal and stressful work environment.

More than once I found myself reacting to situations in ways I would not have anticipated. The insights I gained were revealing and often painful. The struggle to maintain my personal sense of identity and purpose was not easy.

Surviving and Coping: Applying Practical Psychology

In my efforts to maintain a reasonable perspective, I discovered—or more accurately, I reaffirmed—some basic guiding principles. First, I came to view planning as more than a tool for reaching desired organizational goals. In a complex, rapidly changing environment, such as that in the office of mental health, the planning process also yields benefits for the individual doing the planning. I came to view the role of planning as a vehicle for maintaining rational behavior. The exercise of setting objectives and practicing problem-solving and communication skills served as a counterbalance, reducing the possibility of too much influence from such other factors as politics and money.

I also rediscovered the value of initiating mutual support activities. In spite of the constant pressure to produce and the ever-present crisis orientation, it was essential to take time away from production activities to deal with how people were feeling.

Finally, there were some concrete interventions and activities that enabled me to keep an appropriate perspective. For example, it was helpful to have a secretary who reminded me once every few months that I was becoming caught up in the stress patterns of the environment. This gentle but direct confrontation allowed me to step back and observe what I was doing. When successful, I was able to break temporarily the spiraling pattern of frenetic activity and increased agitation. Other homespun remedies included deliberately walking slowly as I traveled throughout the building; maintaining a sense of imagination and humor; and remembering that everyone around me was experiencing the same stresses and conflicts. I found myself continually reminding myself what was important—both personally and professionally. Without this periodic self-coaching, it was easy to lose sight of what was really important and adopt those bureaucratic and politically expedient coping mechanisms that reduce the immediate anxiety but divert one from the substantive issues, problems, and goals of the field.

IN CONCLUSION

As a community psychologist, the experience of working in a central office of state government provided me with a rich opportunity to learn more about the field of mental health, as well as about the work setting. The pace and complexity of that work environment and its relation to the wide array of human services and political subsystems at the federal, state, and local levels were certainly unique. Yet, in the final analysis, I found that this work environment was not essentially different from other community settings. The same organizational development principles and approaches used in other settings were also applicable to the central office environment. And, as in other community settings, anyone interested in creating change would be wise to approach this setting with a fair amount of respect for the strengths of the environmental institutional forces—and humility for one's own ability to have a direct impact on the essential dynamics of the system.

POINTS TO PONDER

1. After reading this chapter, has your view of large government agencies changed? In what way?

2. How would you characterize the state department of mental health described in this chapter in relation to Hargrove and Glidewell's model (see Chapter 2) for classifying the viability of public management jobs? Are there strategies that could have been employed to enhance the legitimacy of that agency's clientele, reduce the intensity of the conflict among constituencies, or otherwise strengthen public confidence in the agency?

3. What organizational approaches or strategies would you employ to enhance the responsiveness of this or other large agencies to the programmatic needs of its consumers?

4. Do any of the personal coping strategies described in this chapter have relevance for your work experience in human services? Are there other coping mechanisms that you find helpful in dealing with the stresses of the work environment?

5. This chapter describes the experience of an individual working in a large state human services agency twenty years ago. Do you think this experience would be different today? In what ways?

CLASSROOM TO COMMUNITY

Applying the Concepts of Change

- Select a human services issue that is currently receiving attention in your local media. From your knowledge of this issue, as well as your readings, identify probable economic, political, social, cultural, technological, and programmatic forces and factors that may be influencing the manner in which this issue is being handled by relevant local, state, and federal agencies. Placing yourself in the role of someone who is interested in promoting particular resolution for this issue, describe the outcome you would like to achieve and the strategies you would employ to deal with the multiple forces that might impact the manner in which this issue is resolved.

Chapter 8

MORE THAN JUST DATA
Evaluating Neighborhood-Based Police Services

Nobody ever said changing human nature was easy.
∼ Charles Grodin, Comedian

T his chapter provides further illustration of the complexity of relationships among parties involved in community programs. Every group from
consumers to politicians to researchers has its own concerns about the implementation and effects of a program. In the situation explored in this chapter,
city police responded to a growing crime rate with a new system. The city
commissioned researchers to evaluate the program, and the results did not
meet their satisfaction. What ensued was a political and ideological struggle.

∼

In 1974 Richard M. Nixon was forced to resign from the presidency of the
United States. Nixon's downfall was brought about by the Watergate incident
and the subsequent cover-up activities of his administration. During this period
in U.S. history, the public lost confidence in the ability of its leaders to govern,
and a pervasive mistrust of elected officials and their appointees developed.

Even in Central New York, far from the fast track of Washington, D.C., an
aura of suspicion pervaded what government officials might do to achieve

their purposes and protect their political interests. As young psychologists involved in evaluating an innovative crime-control project in a midsize Northeastern city, we learned how the political process dealt with the perceived threat. We experienced firsthand the conflicts and anxiety that arise when one is embroiled in a politically charged situation.

THE PROJECT

In 1971 this city of two hundred thousand with a declining industrial base, a prominent university, and a sizeable low-income, inner-city black population instituted an innovative team-policing program in order to reduce crime, enhance community services, and improve relationships with neighborhood residents. In response to widespread concern about growing crime rates and increased hostility toward police, the city created Crime Control Teams (CCT) comprised of specially trained officers assigned to specific geographic sections of the city in order to provide a full range of police services to residents of those areas. Members of these teams were trained to utilize a wide range of skills in order to meet residents' needs for a broad spectrum of police services. The CCT were designed to supplement existing police services in high-crime neighborhoods.

The goal of the program was to reinstate the "cop on the beat" approach by deploying police officers to designated neighborhoods. City officials believed the officers would become familiar with the residents, who in turn would call on members of the neighborhood CCT not only for crime deterrence and intervention but also for other services critical to the safety and well-being of the community.

The federal agency that funded the CCT project required the program to be evaluated by an organization not directly involved in the implementation of the project. The evaluation contract was given to the university research corporation that subcontracted with the Institute for Community Development, a small not-for-profit agency concerned with using social science knowledge and methodology to assist community organizations and agencies. Since one of the principal goals of the CCT project was to improve relationships between police and neighborhood residents, the primary focus of the evaluation was to assess citizen attitudes toward innovative police services.

PLANNING THE EVALUATION

The CCT experiment was, in many ways, a progressive project. The notion of directly involving police officers in community enhancement activities was a radical departure from police practice of that era. In one sense, the

CCT project was a harbinger of today's community policing approach. The initial attitudes of the city government and police department toward program evaluation were also relatively enlightened. Recognizing that program evaluation required comparing the experimental approach with a situation in which CCT concepts were not being implemented, administrators agreed to an evaluation design in which measures would be taken prior to the program's implementation and two years after its inception. The evaluation was to be conducted in the neighborhoods in which team policing was to be practiced as well as in relatively similar neighborhoods in which traditional police practices still existed. Finally, in the spirit of citizen participation, neighborhood residents would be hired and trained to collect evaluation data.

Given the project's emphasis on improving relationships between neighborhood residents and police, it was decided that a survey of citizen attitudes would be used as the principal assessment tool. The survey instrument was designed by the Institute for Community Development and reviewed by representatives of city government and the police department as well as several prominent members of the designated neighborhoods. In addition to identifying demographic characteristics of the respondents, the survey instrument asked neighborhood residents about their attitudes toward, and experience with, police services.

While the collaborative planning among city and police officials, neighborhood leaders, and social scientists was for the most part harmonious and productive, there were two issues that took some effort to resolve. First, the thirteen interviewers recruited from the CCT and control neighborhoods initially objected to the format of the interviews. They felt that the highly structured questions with their fixed-choice response format would restrict the information that could be gathered. They also questioned why demographic identification was required. Lengthy discussions were conducted in which the indigenous interviewers and the researchers enhanced each other's awareness of potential problems of various data-collection approaches. Eventually a survey instrument was created that addressed the concerns of the neighborhood residents while retaining the methodological rigor required to conduct survey research.

The second issue concerned the dissemination of the evaluation results. This matter, which was later to become a major source of contention, arose in response to a previous experience of the consultants in evaluating a program involving the police department. In that project, Institute for Community Development staff, operating under the assumption that data from publicly funded projects should be readily accessible, wanted to disseminate the evaluation results to the public as well as to professionals interested in police services. The program administrators, on the other hand, believed that they should have discretion regarding the release of evaluation data. The debate that ensued focused on questions of public accountability and administrative prerogative. The final resolution represented a compromise that allowed for limited release of results through professional channels but did not meet the researchers' expectation that the results of programs supported by government funds should be made available to the general public.

This earlier conflict heightened the researchers' awareness of the importance of developing an explicit agreement concerning the dissemination of program evaluation results. Since the CCT project required considerable cooperation from neighborhood residents, researchers felt an obligation to return something to the community. Dissemination of the results to the news media and distribution of recommendations to all interested parties, including civic organizations, was viewed as one way of providing payback.

Toward this end the researchers were able to insert into the evaluation contract a clause stating that results of the evaluation would first be submitted to city officials and the police department. After sixty days, the researchers could make this information available to the news media.

IMPLEMENTING THE EVALUATION

The survey instrument was designed to elicit information from neighborhood residents on a number of questions. In addition to collecting data on demographic characteristics of the respondents, the survey included questions in the following areas of concern:

1. Who would you call in a variety of situations, such as a neighbor has a heart attack, you hear gunfire, or you receive an eviction notice?
2. What are your attitudes and feelings about police and police services?
3. How much contact and awareness do you have about police and police services? For example, how often do you talk to police in your neighborhood: never, seldom, sometimes, often, very often.
4. What are your priorities about police services and crime protection, for example, more police, police officers on foot, police serving as coaches for sports activities with youth, crackdown on drug sales?

After pilot-testing a sample of approximately 200 respondents from neighborhoods not involved in the CCT project, the preintervention survey was administered to a stratified sample of 930 persons, with approximately 350 interviews conducted in each CCT area and an additional 200 surveys completed in the control neighborhoods. After the CCT program had been in place for approximately eighteen months, a postsurvey questionnaire was administered to 950 individuals with approximately the same demographic and geographic distribution characteristics as the original sample. Questions asked in the postsurvey were identical to those addressed in the presurvey.

EVALUATION RESULTS

A comparison of the before and after survey responses indicated that residents polled during the postsurvey expressed more positive attitudes toward police than those interviewed during the presurvey. The greatest increase in positive attitudes occurred, however, in the control neighborhoods. This pattern of increasing positive attitudes was found for both black and white respondents, though whites expressed more positive attitudes than blacks at both the beginning and end of the study. The only group that became more negative over time was black teenage males.

Pre- and postcomparisons on specific subsections of this survey yielded the following results:

1. While respondents demonstrated an increased willingness to call police for a variety of concerns at the completion of this study, respondents in the control area expressed an inclination to call police in a wider range of situations than respondents in the experimental districts.

2. No clear relationship was found between the frequency of seeing police in the neighborhoods and attitudes toward police.

3. Respondents who had previous experience in penal institutions or detention homes expressed equally negative attitudes toward police in the before and after periods.

4. CCT residents in control and experimental neighborhoods reported increased awareness of the existence of CCTs during the course of the study.

5. By the end of the study, a small increase was observed in the experimental neighborhoods in the number of residents who indicated that they personally knew police officers, while there was a decrease in reported personal knowledge in the control district.

6. Over the course of the study, a substantial increase was observed within experimental neighborhoods in the number of respondents who endorsed the need for change in police services, while the same endorsement decreased in control neighborhoods.

Taken as a whole the results are, at best, ambiguous. While reported attitudes toward police became more positive in the CCT areas, the increase was not as great as the positive change found in the control area. It was not possible to ascertain from the data whether the shift toward more favorable attitudes was related to departmentwide changes in police practice throughout the city or was due to a societal change in attitudes toward police associated with a more conservative political climate or fewer overt manifestations of social protest.

Although neighborhood respondents' attitudes toward police are not a direct indicator of the effectiveness of neighborhood policing, the results also do not demonstrate that the neighborhood approach is ineffective. In fact, findings such as the increase in personal knowledge of police officers among respondents in the experimental area might be taken as an indication that the project had achieved some of its goals.

Given the absence of unequivocally negative evidence about the effectiveness of the crime-control team program, we were ill-prepared for the reaction we received from police and city officials when we attempted to exercise our contractual prerogative to disseminate the evaluation results.

THE PLOT THICKENS

Our evaluation contract stipulated that the results of the study could be released to the media sixty days after the report had been submitted to the city. As the release date approached, we contacted the university research corporation to inform them of our dissemination plans. Unfortunately, the original project director for this project had died and no one else at the research corporation had been involved with the initial negotiation of the contract. Therefore, when the new project director received our message he decided to discuss our plan with program management staff at city government.

Several days later we received a call from the research corporation project director informing us that the city officials did not want us to release the evaluation results until after the mayoral election, which was to be held in a few months.

Being relatively young and somewhat idealistic, we objected to this directive, stating that we had honored the stipulated sixty-day waiting period and we intended to release the evaluation. A series of unproductive discussions ensued with the research corporation staff attempting to play mediator. While administrators of the research corporation understood our rationale for wanting to make findings of the evaluation study available to the public, they were also aware of the potential political ramifications of publicizing a major crime-control initiative that had not demonstrated increased effectiveness in comparison to traditional practice. In addition to being sensitive to the city administration's perceived vulnerability, the research corporation had a vested interest in maintaining a positive relationship with the city. Given the large amount of federal funding for research-related projects the city received, the research corporation was reluctant to jeopardize its favorable status with the city. Since the research corporation had subcontracted with us, they were concerned that our unwillingness to accede to the request to not release the evaluation report would cause the city to judge them as guilty by association.

Several days before we were scheduled to release the report, the project director of the research corporation called to tell us that we had been invited to a meeting at the office of the chief of police. This news created more than a little anxiety among our small group of researchers. It was one thing to uphold our scientific integrity through a process of three-way communication conducted through the telephone lines and written correspondence. It was quite different to sit face to face with the chief of police who had worked hard to earn a reputation as an intimidating figure.

The reality was worse than the fantasy. The meeting was held in the chief's office. He sat at the end of a U-shaped table flanked by flags of the city, state, and country. Sitting at the table were several city officials as well as representatives of the research corporation. After everyone had been introduced, we engaged in some polite conversation about the project and the issue of releasing the data. Feeling more than a little intimidated by the formidable presence of the police chief, I nonetheless reiterated our reasons for wanting to release the report. The research corporation staff looked uncomfortable and the city officials listened quietly. After a few minutes, the chief turned to me and said that he appreciated our candor in expressing our position and that he intended to be direct and honest with us as well. With that, he said that he was very displeased with our reluctance to accept the city's request not to release the report. He explained that he and city officials did not consider our rationale for disobeying their request to be legitimate. He then told us that he intended to obtain a court injunction restraining us from releasing any information related to the evaluation report. He thanked us for coming to his office and adjourned the meeting.

It would be an understatement to say that we were in a state of high anxiety. Whether it was the intimidating aura of the setting, the toughness of the police chief, or the generally hypersuspicious mood that had been created by the Watergate fiasco, or some combination of these factors, my colleagues and I felt anxious, one might even say paranoid, as we left the meeting.

The next few days were consumed with worrying about what would happen. In the spirit of the times, each of us took a copy of the evaluation report and the contract with its sixty-day dissemination clause and hid them in a place that was unlikely to be discovered by individuals intent on destroying the evidence. We worried about alternative scenarios. What should we do if the injunction were granted? Should we retain a lawyer? Should we hurry to release the report before the chief had a chance to obtain a restraining order? Or would our actions be considered even more flagrant in light of our knowledge of the chief's intention to seek legal recourse? Our anxiety was not helped by the fact that the police chief's brother happened to be a judge in the same city.

ACHIEVING CLOSURE

In the end, cool heads prevailed. After waiting several days without an officer of the court appearing at our doorstep to serve us a restraining order, we prepared a brief news release describing the study and sent it to the local newspapers and radio and television stations. In spite of the absence of any overt or covert attempt to interfere with what we considered to be our right of free speech, we continued to keep copies of the documents in their secret hiding places.

In what we experienced to be an anticlimactic ending, there was no mention of our study in any of the local media for several weeks. One morning, while scanning a local newspaper I almost missed a brief article about our report that was buried on the next to last page of the local news section. The article succinctly summarized the results of the study. There was no comment by city officials, and we were not contacted by reporters before or after the article appeared. As far as we could tell, we might have been the only ones in the city to have read the article.

The mayor won his bid for reelection, CCTs were discontinued, and we were not asked by either the university research corporation or the city administration to conduct any further program evaluation studies.

WHAT WE ACHIEVED AND WHAT WE LEARNED

As researchers venturing into the real world, with all of its complexities, we were not prepared for the resistance we encountered in attempting to share the knowledge gained from our evaluation study. Nor did we know what to do with that knowledge to ensure that it served the purpose for which it was intended. Our principles were righteous, but our strategic skills left something to be desired.

Part of our problem was our lack of clear, realistic expectations about the role of program evaluation and the process of policy formulation and program development. On the most cynical level, program evaluation can be viewed as merely a necessary requisite for receiving funding. A more optimistic perspective is that program evaluation studies and the knowledge derived from them can serve as the driving forces for change. Somewhere in between, and probably more viable, is the view that carefully crafted program evaluation studies and thoughtful interpretation and dissemination of their findings can have a modest, positive influence. Researchers who possess a broad understanding of the political, economic, and social forces that influence policy and program formulation can design and conduct evaluation research that may influence decision makers. The extent of their influence is dependent on the scope of the program being studied and the extent to which key decision makers share the same views about the purpose and goals of the program. As Carol Weiss (1972) observed, the results of program evaluation studies may have a life-or-death impact on small programs within single organizations, whereas the maximum impact an evaluation may have on a large service system is to facilitate minor realignment of system components or tweak some of its support procedures and processes in the direction of greater responsiveness or efficiency.

While it was naive to believe that the results of our study would be embraced enthusiastically by city officials, their receptivity might have been enhanced if we had met with them consistently throughout the project to receive their input and provide them with interim data. We spent considerable time engaging their involvement during the design phase of the project but did not devote much energy to this task during the project's eighteen-month operation. In spite of the awkward manner in which we acted to support our belief that knowledge derived from government-supported research should remain in the public domain, we have no regrets that we behaved in a manner consistent with these principles. In an environment of constant pressure and change it becomes particularly important for social scientists engaged in applied research to maintain an awareness of their ethical and moral responsibilities. One need not adhere blindly to a rigid set of abstract principles in order to behave appropriately. If an applied researcher understands the context in which he or she operates, including the multiple constraints confronting decision makers, research findings are more likely to serve their intended purpose: to inform the decisions of policy makers and administrators.

Perhaps the most important lesson learned is that planning a program evaluation project does not end with the establishment of a research design. Anticipating how the knowledge derived from these studies might be used and what processes and mechanisms can be put in place to ensure that this knowledge reaches receptive ears are equally important facets of the program evaluation process. However, even if we had possessed the foresight to advocate for the establishment of a citizen advisory committee to assist in the design and evaluation of the CCT project, the ultimate fate of the CCT experiment might not have been different. The dilemma of the researchers, finding themselves in the difficult position of being the sole advocates for utilizing research data to inform public policy about police practice might, however, have been averted.

POINTS TO PONDER

1. How would you describe the relationship between the police and the community where you live now or grew up? Do you know of any evaluation of services that has occurred? Do you think such results would have an impact on the community?

2. Can you propose a plan for the researchers that might have avoided such resistance on the part of the research corporation and the city officials?

3. Where do you see the influence of politics in your work with human services organizations?

4. Have you participated in program evaluation of any kind? If so, how were the results used? Did they bring about change? What were the reactions?

5. The beginning of this chapter discusses a particular political moment in the United States. Do you think the distrust of government officials has increased since then? How do you think a request to disseminate results of an evaluation of a community policing intervention might be received today?

CLASSROOM TO COMMUNITY

Applying the Concepts of Change

• As a staff member of a human services agency, you have been asked to report to the board of directors on the progress of a new initiative. You have been working with the agency for several years, but you have worked on this initiative for six months. You know that this project is the executive director's "baby" and that he worked very hard to get the board's approval; however, several major problems in the implementation of this program have manifested. How do you prepare for this meeting with the board of directors? What are your considerations in deciding what and how you will present to the board?

CHAPTER 9

BEYOND RHETORIC
ESTABLISHING A COMPREHENSIVE SERVICES
SYSTEM FOR CHILDREN AND FAMILIES

> *Words are so easy, action is so difficult. To proclaim one's beliefs, to profess one's convictions is one thing; to enact them, to face the hard ugly realities . . . is quite another.*
>
> ⌐ Adlai Stevenson, U.S. Presidential Candidate and
> Ambassador to the United Nations

I f it takes a village to raise a child, what does it take to make a community care for all of its children? Much has been written about the conceptual underpinnings of comprehensive systems of care for children and families, yet few examples of exemplary practice can be found in this area. This chapter describes one state's efforts to develop a comprehensive system of services that is responsive to the needs and strengths of children with emotional and behavioral problems and their families. In this discussion of Virginia's Comprehensive Services Act for At Risk Youth and Families, several critical issues relevant to the establishment of comprehensive services systems are highlighted. The magnitude and complexity of this challenge are underscored through the description of the enormous amount of time and resources required to design the program, enact the enabling legislation, and surmount the obstacles that impeded the transformation of philosophy and theory into practice. The difficulty of achieving an appropriate balance among programmatic, political, and fiscal concerns is also described. Returning to the metaphor of the village, we see how important and difficult it is to shift responsibilities for children and families from the often criticized faceless state and federal bureaucracies traditionally responsible for child and family services to local communities that are vociferous about controlling their own affairs but sometimes appear ambivalent and ill-prepared to assume responsibility for all affected children.

~

Until recently, efforts to improve the delivery of services to children with serious emotional and behavioral difficulties have been long on rhetoric and short on action. Numerous commissions and blue-ribbon panels have concluded that the child service system is woefully inadequate: There are not enough resources to meet the multiple needs of children with emotional and behavioral disturbance, and the resources that exist are disproportionately allocated to pay for highly restrictive and often inappropriate residential services. To make matters worse, the child service delivery system is extremely fragmented and disjointed. The lack of clear roles and responsibilities among child-serving agencies has resulted in poor interagency relationships, nonproductive expenditure of energy and money, and territorial squabbles (Joint Commission on the Mental Health of Children, 1969; President's Commission on Mental Health, 1978; United States Office of Technology Assessment, 1986).

Given the high degree of consensus on what ails the child service system, it seems reasonable to ask why there has been so little progress in improving services for youth. As one might expect, there is no simple answer to this question. One reason for the lag in child services is the low priority that has historically been given to children's mental health. Relatively little funding or energy has been invested in research directed at understanding the causes, prevention, and treatment of children's emotional and behavioral problems. Until the mid 1980s very little systematic research on child mental health services was conducted. Consequently, knowledge and technology about treating emotional and behavioral disturbance among youth are limited.

In addition to lacking state-of-the-art knowledge, insufficient attention has been given to addressing the organizational and fiscal problems associated with providing services to young people. Most children with serious emotional or behavioral problems have multiple needs that include educational, social, and economic as well as health and mental health needs. Traditionally, these needs have been served by categorical agencies such as schools and mental health clinics, each having its own set of eligibility criteria and funding mechanisms. While there has been general agreement that holistic and coordinated service approaches are more likely to be effective, child service administrators, providers, and advocates have had limited success in stream-lining and integrating organizational and funding components of the service system. Difficulties in integrating services for children and families have been further compounded by nonproductive intergovernmental conflict, particularly at the state and local levels. In the absence of sufficient political clout, it has been difficult to overcome the territorial inertia of established bureaucratic systems, even when technically sound plans have been proposed.

In the mid 1980s administrators and researchers began to give serious attention to the question of how to better organize and finance services for children with emotional and behavioral disturbance and their families. In some instances, reform was based on earlier efforts to improve delivery of services to adults. In other cases, efforts in child services have surpassed what has been done for adults, in spite of the fact that the service system for children is inherently more complex. The following account describes one state's ambitious efforts to make the children's service delivery system more responsive to young people and their families. While large system reform efforts do not have actual starting and ending points—they typically proceed in evolutionary fashion—a chronological description of events preceding the actual change is presented in order to illustrate the developmental nature of service system change. The point of departure is selected as arbitrary, corresponding with my entry into this particular child service system.

BUILDING A FOUNDATION FOR CHANGE

Like many other states, in the mid 1980s Virginia had a relatively weak service system for children and adolescents with serious emotional and behavioral problems. In spite of its relatively strong economic and educational base and isolated examples of excellent programs, the overall quality of children's services was not very good. Virginia suffered from many of the same problems in delivering human services as other states: tension between local and state government regarding responsibility for and control of decision making, delivery, and financing; absence of proactive cooperative planning among child-serving agencies; and an over-reliance on the use of hospitalization and residential placement for children experiencing emotional and behavioral difficulties. The lack of a strong, unified constituency on behalf of children further impeded the development of services.

Fortunately, the state commissioner of mental health, who had established a strong community service and support initiative for adults with chronic mental illness, recognized the need to develop a parallel system for children and adolescents. In 1985 he convened a child mental health work group and charged it with developing a blueprint for strengthening children's mental health services in the Commonwealth. Being familiar with a series of previous children's planning reports that served little purpose other than occupying space on a bookshelf, the commissioner exhorted the work group to produce an implementation plan with short- and long-term recommendations for corrective action. The work group—comprised of individuals from various children's mental health constituencies, including the director of the state division for children, a member of the state board of mental health and mental retardation, a private provider, and staff from local and state mental health agencies—took his charge seriously and produced a report that included recommendations and major budget initiatives for child and adolescent community services as well as a detailed set of strategy and policy recommendations for developing a single system of child and adolescent mental health services with appropriate roles and responsibilities for community services boards, state facilities, private providers, and other child-serving agencies.

Until that time, children and adolescents had occupied a relatively low place on the department's priority list. Given the large amount of money and personnel allocated to adult services and the high political profile of the deinstitutionalized population, policy makers and administrators spent most of their time dealing with crises in the adult service delivery system. As a result, little attention was given to the mental health needs of children, adolescents, and their families.

In what later proved to be a prophetic event, the commissioner of mental health, shortly before leaving his position to accept a similar post in another state, called a press conference to announce the work group's findings and recommendations. Standing before the television cameras, he explained that while the development of community services for adults who are seriously mentally ill had been the number-one priority of the department for the past decade, it was time to undertake a major new initiative. He articulated the department's commitment to youth with serious emotional disturbances and outlined a series of policy and program development activities that would be undertaken to improve services for children and families.

In spite of the commissioner's strong statement of support, child advocates remained skeptical. First, they were not convinced that the commissioner's replacement would adopt the same agenda. More important, their awareness of the importance of interagency collaboration in effectively meeting children's needs and the formal impediments that existed in this area raised doubt about how effective a single agency's initiative might be in addressing problems of children's services. Over the course of the next eight years, a series of activities—some intentionally planned, but many simply fortuitous—culminated in the creation of an innovative statewide system of care for troubled youth and their families. The accomplishment of this feat surprised even the most ardent skeptics.

BREAKING THE MOLD

Consistent with other major reforms, the establishment of a comprehensive system of services for at risk youth and their families cannot be attributed to a single individual or event. There were, however, several critical activities that enabled the Commonwealth to alter some of its fundamental service delivery, fiscal, and organizational patterns that had historically served as impediments to responding effectively to the needs of youth with emotional and behavioral problems and their families. The most notable pivotal events, which occurred between 1986 and 1993, include the following.

Involvement of the Commonwealth's First Lady The 1985 election not only brought into office a governor with strong interest in mental health; it also yielded a first lady with a long-term commitment to literacy who was looking for opportunities to play a constructive role in improving services to young people. Sensing the activist orientation of the first lady, several child advocates invited her to participate in the child mental health arena. Initially, the first lady agreed to become honorary chair of the advisory committee of the Virginia Treatment Center for Children, the state's leading public child mental health facility. Serving in this capacity enabled the first lady to heighten her awareness of the major issues and problems in providing effective services to children and families. She was particularly concerned with the disjointed and territorial manner in which state child-serving agencies related to each other and expressed an interest in doing something to remedy that situation. When she was approached with the proposal that she convene a forum of policy makers, providers, and consumers to address this issue, she immediately accepted.

To prepare for this event, several small interagency work groups drafted position papers describing problems and possible solutions in areas such as early intervention and prevention services, and interagency coordination. Because of the first lady's influence, most of the significant state-level policy makers attended the forum. The participants included cabinet-level secretaries responsible for education, juvenile justice, and health and human services as well as the commissioners for all of the major child-serving agencies. After hearing a keynote address and planning committee reports, the cabinet secretaries and agency heads were given an opportunity to respond. Finally, the first lady addressed the panel of top state officials.

In her presentation, the first lady challenged the cabinet secretaries to work with their agencies to identify and implement creative, efficient ways to improve the coordination of children's services among state and local agencies. She asked them specifically to develop a plan for achieving interagency coordination, including organizational and fiscal mechanisms that would allow children with serious emotional and behavioral problems to receive services tailored to their unique unmet needs without having to experience bureaucratic frustrations and delays. She closed her remarks by asking the secretaries to report their progress to her in six months.

Small Steps in the Right Direction   Deliberations of the cabinet secretaries, agency heads, and their staff led to the establishment of the State Interagency Consortium on Child Mental Health. The consortium, comprised of a board of state agency staff, local providers, and family members, initiated two funding programs designed to facilitate collaborative provision of community-based services. Both of these initiatives were supported by funds that each state child-serving agency contributed to a common resource bank administered by the consortium. Separating these funds from the jurisdiction of individual agencies permitted greater flexibility in responding to child and family needs. Initial allocation of funds to the consortium was $1.6 million. This money was used to fund two new initiatives:

• *The State Interagency Funds Pool.*   Local communities were invited to apply for small grants to support individualized programs for children whose service needs could not be met within the existing regulatory constraints using available resources. In order to ensure that agencies were working collaboratively, the consortium required the directors of local social service, mental health, education, and other relevant child-serving agencies to provide written verification of involvement of all agencies and family members in development of the service plan.

• *Local Interagency Service Projects.*   Recognizing that many communities had critical gaps in their continuum of care, the consortium solicited proposals from localities for the development of coordinated service delivery approaches that created new services that connected to current services. Localities were required to demonstrate that child-serving agencies would jointly plan and operate these programs. Through a competitive award process, six localities were given up to $200,000 each for local interagency service demonstration projects.

During the next three years, localities submitted 245 requests to the funds pool to supplement service plans for individual children. Each year the percentage of applications approved for funding increased, with 52 percent of proposals accepted between 1988 and 79 percent approved in 1990. The type of service requested during this period also shifted. Initially, requests for residential group care comprised slightly more than 50 percent of the applications. By 1990, only 21 percent were requests for residential group care, with the remainder focused on smaller homelike settings and other community services (MacBeth, 1993).

***Creating a Critical Interagency Linkag**e*   During the mid to late 1980s, organizations at both the local and state levels moved closer to establishing coordinated, comprehensive services for at risk youth. While some of these efforts were strictly at the cognitive level, with agency personnel becoming more familiar with basic concepts and engaging in discussion about collaboration, concrete examples of constructive action also were evident, as illustrated by the number of applications made to the interagency consortium.

One particularly significant initiative, though largely unanticipated, occurred at the state policy board level. Each of Virginia's state agencies is governed by a board of citizens appointed by the governor. These boards are vested with the authority to establish and approve agency policies. In some instances, these boards have functioned as a rubber stamp, endorsing a commissioner's recommendations. In other cases, activist boards have been responsible for establishing major changes in policy.

The board of the Virginia State Department of Mental Health, Mental Retardation, and Substance Abuse Services decided to play an active role in enhancing cooperation among child-serving agencies. At the suggestion of one of its members, a woman who had served on the commissioner's child mental health work group and had been involved in the planning of the first lady's forum, the board invited other state child-serving agency boards to join with them in establishing a joint board liaison committee for children's services. The purpose of this liaison group was to share information about activities in respective agencies and to develop strategies on how to strengthen collaborative efforts on behalf of at risk youth and families. In addition to generating constructive suggestions and participating in various interagency planning activities, the mere presence of this group served as a reminder to agency heads that genuine collaboration among agencies was an important priority.

OTHER POSITIVE INFLUENCES

During this period of time, several other streams of activity converged to support the development of a coordinated approach to serving children and families. PACCT (Parents and Children Coping Together), which was established in 1985 after a statewide conference on developing partnerships between parents and professionals, received assistance from the federal Child and Adolescent Service System Program (CASSP), which was designed to stimulate service system development at the state level. Through CASSP, which provided seed money as well as a conceptual framework for developing integrated systems of care for children and adolescents with mental health problems, PACCT received grant funds to strengthen family network activities at the local and state level.

This multifaceted approach, including activity at the grassroots, service-provider, and state-policy levels, succeeded in realigning the orientation for children's services in Virginia. Although these activities were not sufficient to achieve a comprehensive system reform, these shifts in perspective and interaction within the child-serving community challenged traditional patterns of behavior and created receptivity for another series of events that would have a significant impact on the course of the service delivery system for the next few years.

HELP COMES FROM AN UNLIKELY SOURCE

In 1988, the State Department of Planning and Budget (DPB), concerned about the rapidly rising cost of residential treatment programs for youth with emotional or behavioral problems, initiated a large-scale study to gain a better understanding of the nature and extent of publicly funded residential care for children and youth. In an investigation of unprecedented magnitude, the DPB tracked every child with emotional or behavioral problems who had spent more than thirty days in a group residential care setting that had been paid for by at least one public agency during fiscal year 1989. The results of the DPB research surprised even seasoned veterans of the child-serving community.

Even after taking into account children with multiple placements during the year, an unduplicated count was tallied of 4,993 young people with emotional or behavioral problems who spent more than thirty days in a group residential care setting or state institution, such as a state psychiatric hospital or corrections facility. While the majority of these youth were placed in programs within the state, more than 300 were in residential programs outside of the Commonwealth. Nearly half of the youngsters had two or more placements during the year; four out of five were involved in two or more agencies, and nearly one of five had contact with four agencies. The incidence of serious and emotional problems was high—nearly 90 percent; more than three-quarters had major school-related problems; and two-thirds had been adjudicated by the courts (Virginia Department of Planning and Budget, 1990).

Perhaps the most striking finding was the cost associated with placement in residential care. During fiscal year 1989, the cost for serving the nearly 5,000 children placed in residential settings was $93.6 million. In fiscal year 1990, this cost rose to $101 million (Virginia Department of Planning and Budget, 1990).

While the primary purpose of the DPB study was to highlight the enormous fiscal burden of residential care for the Commonwealth, this research project had an important secondary purpose—one might even say benefit. The study team spent considerable time speaking to experts in child services in order to gain a better understanding of the current system. In its final report, the DPB described a strategy for achieving programmatic and financial goals that was remarkably similar to the approach that the child-serving community had advocated for the past several years. The combination of the DPB's influential position within state government and the perception that the state's chief fiscal agency clearly did not have a vested interest in a particular approach to service delivery gave the DPB study a measure of credibility that might not have existed if it had been conducted by an organization associated with children's causes.

AN AMBITIOUS PLANNING PROCESS

The results of the residential-care study elicited considerable interest within the executive and legislative branches of state government. In response to the general assembly's mandate that a detailed implementation plan be developed that addressed all of the children's residential-services study recommendations, the governor created the Council on Community Services for Youth and Families to implement fundamental structural and functional changes in the current system. The council, which reported directly to the three cabinet secretaries responsible for children's services, undertook a comprehensive planning process, unprecedented for the scope of its mission and the scope and diversity of activity participants. The 145 council members, comprised of public and private service providers, parents, child advocates, university personnel, judges, local government officials, and state agency personnel, were assigned to work groups charged with developing detailed plans for establishing and implementing a comprehensive system of services for at risk youth and their families. The work groups addressed issues such as designing a model of community services, establishing funding mechanisms, and creating a local interagency process. Council work groups also focused on training, technical assistance and utilization review, tracking, and evaluation. A work group also oversaw five local demonstration projects funded by a two-year $2.4 million appropriation from the state general assembly.

During the next eighteen months, the council and its work groups discussed alternative approaches to developing, operating, and supporting a comprehensive system of care. The challenge of designing a system that would meet the needs of the multiple constituents involved in children's services quickly became apparent as the work groups struggled to reach consensus. While it would be an exaggeration to claim that the council achieved full agreement on all of the issues it addressed, when the time came to submit a report to the governor, the group had developed and endorsed a comprehensive plan for serving children and families. Following are the objectives of the proposed service delivery system (Virginia Acts of Assembly, Chapter 880, Section 2.1-745):

- Ensure that services and funding are consistent with the Commonwealth's policy goals of preserving families and providing appropriate services in the least restrictive environment, while protecting the welfare of children and maintaining the safety of the public;
- Identify and intervene early with young children and their families who are at risk of developing emotional or behavioral problems or both due to environmental, physical, or psychological stress;
- Increase interagency collaboration and family involvement in service delivery and management;
- Encourage a public and private partnership in the delivery of services; and
- Provide communities flexibility in the use of funds and to direct decisions, authority, and accountability to communities who know best the needs of their youth and families.

Unlike many large-scale proposals, this plan did not compromise the vision and values that had been established initially in order to achieve consensus. The proposed system of care was innovative and bold. Funding would be shifted from categorical programs controlled by state agencies to local resource pools with the flexibility to be used to support service programs tailored to the unique needs of each child and family. In each locality, multidisciplinary committees comprised of agency representatives and family members—Family Assessment and Planning Teams—would work collaboratively to assess needs and strengths of the family and to design individualized service programs to meet these needs. Responsibility and authority for the system of care would be clearly vested with each locality rather than with the state. At the state level, multiple existing interagency teams would be consolidated into a single structure that would be responsible for coordinating program and fiscal policies, supporting community efforts, and reducing duplication and fragmentation of state requirements across agencies. Provision was made to support communities' interests in developing early intervention services for at risk children and their families.

Why was Virginia able to succeed in translating the theoretical concepts underpinning responsive community-based services into a viable program proposal accompanied by appropriate organizational and financing mechanisms? How did the program initiators gain the support of the state executive branch as well as constituents interested in child services? What variables differentiated the Commonwealth of Virginia from many other states that had addressed this issue but failed to reach acceptable resolution? While one of the answers to all these questions is that Virginia acted more swiftly than other states that would eventually follow similar courses of action, some specific factors account for Virginia's success. Certainly the early support of the commissioner of the Department of Mental Health, Mental Retardation, and Substance Abuse Services, the state boards, and the first lady facilitated the initial developmental activity that led to the council's planning efforts. The Department of Mental Health's Work Group on Child Adolescent Services, the First Lady's Forum, and the State Interagency Consortium tested concepts and strategies that would later be incorporated into the council's proposal. Other forces, however, accounted for the successful collaborative effort, including the following:

1. *The constructive role of the Secretary of Health and Human Services.* Every major reform effort requires a leader who will advocate for and guide the initiative through its precarious course of development. In the case of the Comprehensive Services Act, the secretary of Health and Human Services played this role quite effectively. Fortunately, this individual previously had been the deputy commissioner and then the commissioner of the State Department of Mental Health during the program's formative period. When the commissioner of mental health who had convened the initial work group first announced that children were to be the department's priority and then left for another position, the deputy commissioner was promoted to the position of commissioner. Initially, he did not have a pronounced interest in children. However, as he became familiar with the issues and incremental progress was made, his commitment to children grew stronger. When the new governor appointed him as secretary of health and human services after he successfully orchestrated a collaborative effort to increase the department's community-based funding, the new secretary announced that the development of a comprehensive, coordinated service delivery system for children and adolescents would be one of his highest priorities.

The secretary's role in developing the proposed children's service system went well beyond merely identifying this initiative as a priority. Using his proven administrative and political skills, he designed a planning process that addressed all substantive issues related to designing a successful system and included representation from every concerned constituent group. Particularly critical was his involving key staff and members of the state organizations representing city and county government. In the final stages of negotiation, when sensitive financial and political matters were being discussed, involvement of these two key organizations made the difference between having the proposal tossed aside and being given careful scrutiny as a potential solution to a serious community problem.

The secretary's constructive influence is exemplified in the manner in which the issue of local control was addressed. Not only did the proposed Comprehensive Services Act remove control of funding from state agencies and place authority for spending decisions with local government, but it also empowered localities to make decisions about the types and volume of services that were most appropriate for each community. The act defined a core group of youth for whom services were mandated and presented a broad menu of potential services to be offered, but it left to each local community the task of assessing its needs and deciding how it would allocate resources. Contrary to the state's conventional position that centralization of authority was required to ensure that all individuals in need of services would receive equitable treatment throughout the state, the secretary advocated for stronger local governance. Without this provision, it is likely that the proposal would not have received endorsement from the key local officials whose support was essential for legislative approval.

2. The cohesive teamwork of the agency heads.   In spite of the almost universal rhetorical support for improving coordination among agencies, this goal has seldom been achieved at the federal, state, or local level. Agency heads often find themselves in the position of trying to reconcile conflict between wanting to build a better system for providing services and responding to the pressure applied by their superiors to deal with day-to-day crises and reduce political vulnerability of the agency and executive branch. Not surprisingly, the political agenda almost always prevails.

In the case of the Comprehensive Services Act, the heads of the major child-serving agencies decided early in the process to meet on a regular basis to discuss critical issues related to the planning process as well as to keep abreast of the council's activities. During the entire eighteen months of the planning process, agency heads met for an hour-and-a-half breakfast meeting every other week. Their discussions were frank and intense. Occasionally they focused on broad conceptual and philosophical issues, trying to develop a rational and coherent framework for the proposed system; however, most of their time was spent formulating pragmatic strategies to address the multiple administrative and political issues included in successfully developing a responsive system of services. In the course of their deliberations, the agency heads' commitment to the comprehensive system grew, and they established an alliance in which they were able to put aside many of the parochial interests of their individual agencies in order to construct a coordinated system of care for children and families.

In addition to providing strong leadership for the council's activities, the unified action of the agency directors had other positive benefits. By demonstrating cooperative and goal-directed behavior, the agency heads served as positive role models for members of their staff involved in various work groups. The trickle-down impact of this collaboration yielded a productive and efficient planning process in which difficult issues were addressed rather than avoided, territorial disputes were kept to a minimum, and proactive problem-solving behavior prevailed.

3. *Paying sufficient attention to detail.* One of the distinguishing features of the council's planning process was the amount of energy devoted to the numerous operational components of a comprehensive services system. The work groups, with their heterogeneous memberships, conducted research on other systems, analyzed relevant data, and spent considerable time discussing alternative approaches until consensus was reached. At times, participants became frustrated with the length and complexity of the process. Although the planning process was cumbersome and time-consuming, it produced a comprehensive, detailed blueprint for creating an innovative system of care for youth with serious emotional and behavioral disturbances and their families. The scope and sophistication of the plan were matched by the degree of acceptance among the council's membership. While every participant did not fully endorse all aspects of the plan, these stakeholders, for the most part, supported the proposal and felt pride of ownership in the council's final report. The endorsement of the plan by its membership was important not only as an indicator of consensus among its designers; many of the council members served as representatives of larger interest groups and became active promoters of the plan among their constituents.

4. *The involvement and support of the Department of Planning and Budget (DPB).* Having served as an impetus for formation of the Governor's Council on Community Service for Youth and Families, the DPB continued to play a vital role as the developmental work proceeded. Budget staff provided

critical technical assistance in analyzing fiscal data and formulating financial mechanisms. As these staff became involved, their investment in the project grew and they eventually became strong supporters and advocates of the proposed service system. In this rare instance of cost-containment goals being compatible with service-improvement initiatives, support by DPB became a critical ingredient in the acceptance by the highest levels of government of the comprehensive services system proposal.

5. *The paradoxical effect of the state's fiscal crisis on the reform of children's services.* Ironic as it may seem, the fact that the state was facing a $2.1 billion shortfall during the period of the council's activity actually may have enhanced its probability of succeeding. The governor, who was the first elected black governor in the United States, considered himself a socially progressive and fiscally conservative Democrat. His cabinet and agency-head appointments were, for the most part, experienced administrators with strong management skills and commitment to service reform. Given the difficult and painful task of dismantling many of the state's popular programs in order to balance the budget, the children's service system initiative, which had a relatively modest price tag attached to it, was viewed as a constructive diversion from the cutback activities and represented the administration's only hope for leaving a positive legacy in the area of human services.

LEAPING THE LAST HURDLE

Among veterans of the child service system, there was a sense of amazement, even disbelief, about the successful planning process of the council. The degree to which the actual plan matched the council's vision, its specificity, and the broad base of support it had received from all constituents were unprecedented. The prevailing attitude within the child-serving community was "this is too good to be true." Unfortunately, the subsequent actions of the legislature would give child advocates reason to believe that this maxim was true.

As one might expect, the issue that altered—at least temporarily—the council's momentum was the proposed methodology for allocating funds. The council's funding work group had struggled with the question of how to distribute state pool funds to localities. Historically, no uniform guidelines had been established for determining funding levels for localities. The amount of money a community had available for children's services depended on a number of factors, including utilization rates, the ability of localities to advocate for state agency funds, funding formulas that required localities to contribute a proportional match to receive state dollars—that is, 10 percent local,

90 percent state contribution—and, most important, the amount of local money the community was willing to spend on children's services.

The funding work group decided that a more rational and consistent methodology was needed to allocate state pool funds. After reviewing many alternatives, the group chose a two-factor formula to assess need and determine allocation levels. The first factor was population. The greater the number of youth in a city or county, the larger their allocation would be. After reviewing the literature, the work group concluded that the level of poverty that existed in a community was the best indicator of need. Low income predicted, as well or better than any other combination of factors, the risk level for youth and families in a given community.

Despite the rational basis for this needs-assessment approach, and its endorsement by local government member representatives on the council, the allocation formula encountered strong opposition from many localities. Since the economic problems of the state precluded authorization of additional funds for children's services because existing agency funds had been unencumbered and their redistribution to local government inevitably would result in a shift in the amount allocated to each locality, application of the reallocation formula, with its reliance on poverty level as a determinant of need, would result in poorer communities receiving an increase in their funding base and richer communities experiencing a relative decline in resources. Anticipating that wealthier communities would react negatively to the loss of revenue they received, the council proposed that an additional $4.8 million be allocated to ensure that no localities would have to provide more local funds in order to maintain their current level of services as they implemented the new funding formula. This hold-harmless provision would gradually be phased out over several years. The group that formulated the hold-harmless provision believed that the maintenance of current funding levels and the incremental approach to redistribution of funds would make this proposal palatable to the legislature. This was not to be the case.

Several wealthy localities mobilized an aggressive campaign to convince legislators to vote against the proposed service reform bill. These localities were joined by a vocal group of local child-serving agency directors interested in preserving their current control of financial resources. Legislators, experiencing difficulty comprehending all facets of this complex act and feeling pressure from some of their constituents, decided to proceed cautiously. They approved provisionally the concept of the Comprehensive Services Act and instructed the governor to continue planning efforts, especially in the area of reallocation methodology, but they postponed action on the funding mechanism until the following year's general assembly session. Advocates for the proposed comprehensive services system were disappointed that a small vocal faction could thwart progress. Their disappointment did not, however, interfere with their commitment to child services reform and they rededicated themselves to refining the plan and advocating on its behalf.

The following year, the governor's staff presented to the legislature a revised formula, using a different measure of poverty and adding to the needs-assessment formula a measure of youth in the community placed out of home. This modification of the allocation formula, along with a more generous hold-harmless provision that reduced the risk of wealthier communities receiving less funding, was sufficient to overcome previous opposition. The legislature, satisfied with the changes in the funding formula and having had an opportunity to better understand and assimilate the operational details of the plan, enacted legislation that would radically change the manner in which children's services were organized, paid for, and delivered in Virginia. In July 1993, localities throughout the state began to implement the Comprehensive Services Act (CSA) for at risk youth and families.

AFTER THE ACT

Shortly after implementation began, it became evident that some children and families were benefitting from the new system. Adolescents who previously might have been sent to residential treatment facilities for extended periods of time were able to remain at home, or at least in their communities, while receiving needed services. In some communities, the degree of family involvement increased noticeably at the direct-service and policy-making levels. Service providers began to restructure their program offerings to be more compatible with the individualized, community-based orientation of the CSA. Examples of creative, flexible funding to meet the needs of families with children who had serious emotional and behavioral problems could be found in several localities.

While supporters of the act were pleased to see these signs of progress, their initial enthusiasm was tempered by enhanced awareness of how difficult it is to actualize a major reform. Although the CSA altered the organizational funding structures of the services system, the passage of this legislation did not ensure successful resolution of operational issues, nor did it bring about fundamental changes in personal and professional orientation required to function in a manner consistent with the basic principles of the act. Paradoxically, the successful resolution of one set of problems sometimes brought to the surface other impediments that had been masked by the attention given to the more blatant problems. For instance, the lack of coordination of services and inflexibility of use of funds created by structural fragmentation of agencies were such strong barriers no compelling reasons could be found to focus on more subtle problems such as the failure of providers to function in a family-friendly manner because of the inadequacy of their own professional preparation. Finally, the internal dynamics of the system and changes in political and social perspectives at the local and state levels also affected the system's course in development. The problems encountered in implementing the Comprehensive Services Act included the following:

• The Comprehensive Services Act's strong emphasis on local autonomy enabled cities and counties to design service systems that met the unique needs of each community. While this increased flexibility made it easier for many children and families to receive better services, it also created new problems for others. Before the Comprehensive Services Act was implemented, each child-serving agency had defined responsibilities for specific populations. Due to resource limitations, these agencies were not always able to fully meet the needs of these designated populations, but in most instances responsibilities were delineated for each agency. Within the Comprehensive Services Act framework, communities were able to define, within limits, priority populations to be served by the Family Assessment and Planning Teams. As responsibility for service shifted to these teams, individual agencies whose resources had been reallocated to the Comprehensive Services Act process narrowed the scope of whom they would serve directly with their reduced resource capacity. Subsequently, many families with children who were not considered priority populations by the local Family Assessment and Planning Teams and who no longer met the individual agencies' criteria for inclusion found themselves ineligible to receive services.

• Passage of the Comprehensive Services Act was accompanied by considerable attention and publicity. The high visibility of the new service delivery system attracted additional referrals. Since the resource base did not increase significantly, many communities found themselves in the position of experiencing greater demand without having the capacity to meet additional requests for services. The increased discrepancy between supply and demand heightened the frustration of families, providers, and policy makers.

• Communities that had been involved in pilot projects associated with the Comprehensive Services Act or that had undertaken service integration initiatives on their own were better prepared to adapt to the new service system. Other communities either did not have an adequate understanding of how to implement the act or preferred the old system. In such instances, staff sometimes voiced rhetorical support for the program but did not behave in a manner consistent with the principles of the act. For instance, one of the major tenets of the act was that staff developing individual service plans should take into account the strengths and needs of the child and family and should actively encourage and promote involvement of family members in the planning process. Even though the formats of service planning meetings were modified to incorporate multiagency participation and flexible funding, many communities still excluded parents from these sessions and continued to operate in a parent-blaming, deficit-oriented mode.

• Although the Comprehensive Services Act had survived—one might even say benefitted from—the state's fiscal crisis of the early 1990s, the system did not fare as well initially under the administration of the next governor, a conservative Republican who campaigned successfully on a "cut spending and lower taxes" platform. All of the cabinet members and agency heads who had become ardent supporters of the act were replaced by new individuals. The "reduce government" mentality translated to less support for human services, both programmatically and financially. The comprehensive services system was still in a relatively early and precarious stage of development. Without strong leadership, many of the critical issues needing resolution went unattended, and some individuals expressed fears that the act would be revoked. This void in support and confidence not only hampered the system's development; it also provided an opportunity for communities that did not have a strong commitment to regress to former practices. In some localities, agencies actually abandoned collaborative planning and funding activities and reverted to a territorial approach in which each agency acted autonomously, devoting more effort to protecting resource bases than to ensuring that families received appropriate services.

LOOKING AHEAD

Considering the dramatic shift in political perspective and the inevitable rejection of the former administration's favorite projects by the new governor, the comprehensive services system's current status was relatively healthy. The original resource base had not been reduced, and additional funds were provided to support growth in the number of children being served. With the turnover of agency heads, an initial absence of cohesive leadership occurred; yet there was no attempt to dismantle the newly created structure. Family members, providers, and administrators in the field continued to grapple with unresolved issues and procedural problems inherent in such a complex system. However, their sophistication and confidence continued to grow as they gained experience working in a collaborative mode.

While it is not possible to predict the long-term outcome of the services system generated by the Comprehensive Services Act, it is reasonable to assume that its course of development will be shaped by the predominant political, social, and economic forces it encounters in the future as well as the internal merits of the program. Just as the evolving chain of events of the past decade laid the groundwork for the creation of this act, the continued growth of the program will be dependent upon the support it receives during the next few years. The vision of the comprehensive services system for children and families would not have been actualized without the strong leadership and advocacy of specific individuals such as the first lady of Virginia, the secretary of health and human services who had formerly served as commissioner of mental health, and the agency heads who coalesced into a productive work group. The surprising convergence of interests, such as the budget division's concern for cost containment and the child advocates' desire to strengthen community services, also played a facilitative role in the establishment of the Comprehensive Services Act. Finally, the perseverance and hard work of a large coalition of providers, administrators, and family members generated detailed guidelines and procedures required to implement this complex system. These groups, who had historically been in conflict with each other, set aside their differences in order to focus on shared values and goals related to improving services for children and families.

As the Comprehensive Services Act entered its second generation of administrative leadership at the state level, it received widespread recognition that its continued success was dependent upon the ability of new individuals and organizations to fill the leadership void. Advocacy would be needed at the grassroots level as well as higher levels of local and state government. A considerable gap still existed between the rhetoric of the act and local communities' actual acceptance of responsibility for serving children and families. This lack of ownership was exacerbated by the current political philosophy, which was more favorable to incarceration than treatment and rehabilitation. Creative leadership would be required to articulate and promote the Comprehensive Services Act goals in a manner that did not jeopardize its survival within the current conservative political and social climate.

Leadership would also be needed to ensure, at the state level, continued viability of the act. Ingenuity would be required to ensure continued interest and support from the executive and legislative branches. One of the hazards of a decentralized approach is the potential loss of state involvement and support that accompanies the shift to local empowerment. Governors and legislators have often withdrawn financial support from important program areas once the locus of authority has moved to local government.

In an era in which less government was considered to be better, the Comprehensive Services Act faced a critical challenge: Could the empowerment of local communities and ultimately individual families be accomplished within a political context in which elected leaders were afraid to be identified as advocates of government support for human services?

When the former secretary of health and human services convened the Governor's Council on Community Services, he told the assembled members that the creation of a comprehensive services system would require that individuals in leadership positions, particularly agency heads, would have to meet together at the planning table, push their financial resources to the center of the table, and then withdraw their hands, leaving the money on the table. As the new system struggled through its infancy, advocates of the Comprehensive Services Act hoped that leaders, at both state and local levels, would not leave the table, taking their support with them.

Fortunately, new leadership emerged to guide the Comprehensive Services Act through its next phase of development. As we see in Chapter 10, however, the problems the young system faced and the direction it took were strongly influenced by the emerging and dominant political and economic forces of that period.

POINTS TO PONDER

1. The concept of a system of services that is integrated programmatically, organizationally, and fiscally has been discussed for a long time. What do you consider to be the principal factors that contributed to the actualization of this concept in Virginia? What advice would you give to another group interested in developing a comprehensive system of care?

2. The issue of how to allocate centralized funding to localities became controversial during the final phase of establishing the Comprehensive Services Act and, in fact, delayed passage of the act for a year. Given the pivotal role of funding in service system reform, innovative approaches to creating fiscal structures and incentives that support program and goals are essential. Are there fiscal approaches that would facilitate service reform initiatives such as the Comprehensive Services Act?

3. The critical role of stakeholders and constituencies within the human services system, particularly regarding the difficulties in reconciling conflicts among these individuals and groups, has been discussed throughout this book. Designers of the Comprehensive Services Act chose to involve a wide range of interested parties in the planning of the comprehensive services system. They realized that a process involving a planning council of 145 members would be challenging, but they believed that if a consensus could be built the chances of the new system succeeding would increase significantly. Do you think this strategy was effective? Are there other viable approaches that might be worth considering in achieving large-scale reform?

4. Creating systems reform is a daunting challenge. What personal characteristics are important for a person in a leadership position who is attempting to shepherd this type of reform initiative?

5. Many significant changes are precipitated by crises. In the case of the Comprehensive Services Act, the dramatic rise in the cost of residential treatment services triggered the involvement of the state department of planning and budget. One wonders if the service system spawned by the Comprehensive Services Act would have been established if this powerful agency had not been involved. Can you site other examples of how crisis situations could be utilized to promote constructive change?

6. A fundamental premise of the Comprehensive Services Act is that children will be better served if localities accept responsibility—or "ownership"—for the care of children and families in need of service. Based on your readings and experience, can you suggest practical strategies that will increase the likelihood of community ownership?

CLASSROOM TO COMMUNITY

Applying the Concepts of Change

- Select a human services system that you are familiar with. Using the principles and goals of the Comprehensive Services Act, assess how well your identified services system adheres to the act's philosophy and achieves its desired outcomes. Describe strategies that you would employ to make this system more responsive to the needs of its consumers.

CHAPTER 10

DEMOCRACY MEETS THE BOTTOM LINE
CARING FOR CHILDREN AND
MANAGING RESOURCES

But visions are never the sole property of one man or one woman.
Before a vision can become a reality, it must be owned by every
single member of the group.

— Phil Jackson, Former Head Coach of the Chicago Bulls

O ne of the most formidable challenges confronting human services
proponents is how to achieve a reasonable balance between providing
appropriate, responsive services and controlling costs in an environment of
scarce resources. Although no proven methods exist for achieving this delicate balance, several promising approaches do. This chapter contains a
description of a statewide initiative to improve services for children with
emotional and behavioral problems while also being responsive to the
demands of cost containment. By employing a multistrategy approach that
relied heavily on input from service system users and other stakeholders,
leadership was able to address the need to develop rational child and family
services assessment and planning processes. These processes were embodied
with a flexible framework that provided considerable opportunities for
localities to tailor the assessment and planning approaches they used to the
unique needs and characteristics of their local communities.

~

Currently, managed care pervades many aspects of everyday life. Discussions of this subject rarely occur without eliciting strong emotional responses. In fact, one might say that "dispassionate deliberation of managed care" is an oxymoron.

Consumers, especially those seeking health-care services, are concerned about shrinking access to traditionally available health-care services as well as decreasing availability of health-care benefits. Health-care and other human-services professionals worry about the impact of cost containment on personal financial status as well as the fiscal well-being of organizations and agencies with which they are affiliated. Providers are also concerned about the impact of managed care on their ability to provide services they believe are needed by their patients or clients. Administrators and government officials struggle to reconcile competing and often conflicting pressures. The public outcry over rising taxes and the cost of health care has driven policy makers and administrators on a cutback crusade while another sector of the population complains vigorously about the declining access to, and quality of, health and human services.

Human services professionals have at least a dual stake in this issue. In our vocational capacity, we are concerned about the well-being of those we serve as well as the continued viability of our livelihood. As citizens, we are acutely aware of the negative impact that may result from cost-containment activities. A recent personal experience illustrates the dilemma posed by these conflicting forces. My father, who had experienced serious complications from vascular surgery, was scheduled to be discharged from the hospital. Because the operation had significantly diminished his ability to care for himself, other members of our family and I were concerned about his safety and worried that he would be at risk if he were discharged from the hospital. Knowing that third-party payors were pushing hospitals to discharge patients quickly, we pleaded with his physicians to keep him in the hospital until he was stabilized and we could make arrangements to care for him appropriately.

The next day I was scheduled to make a presentation on a study we were conducting to test the feasibility of applying utilization management tools to a statewide comprehensive services system for children with serious emotional and behavioral disorders and their families. The purpose of this study was to examine methods for controlling costs and ensuring that children who could be served in homelike, community-based service settings would not inappropriately be placed in residential treatment programs. While the leadership of the Comprehensive Services Act had emphatically stressed the importance of providing services appropriate to the needs and strengths of the child and family and retaining decision-making authority at the local level, it was also apparent that controlling the cost of the program must be a primary objective of any utilization management adopted for the act.

As I thought about my utilization management presentation, following on the heels of my recent experience trying to extend my father's hospital stay, I became aware of the differences in how I approached these two events. Initially, I was struck by the apparent contradiction in my position. How could I advocate so strongly for extending my father's hospital stay, knowing the high cost of acute inpatient care, while, at the same time, arguing that we must restrict the use of residential treatment for children with serious emotional and behavioral problems? Was I being hypocritical, advocating for more expensive care while at the same time lecturing to others about why they should not overutilize high levels of care when service could be provided in a less restrictive setting? Or was I taking the economically prudent side of this argument because it was the politically correct thing to do and would ensure continuation of my services as a consultant?

Upon further reflection, I realize that my initial reaction was based on an oversimplification of the issues and that, as with most complex social issues, any unidimensional solution would be insufficient and probably less than honest. Reaching this conclusion did not relieve me entirely of my internal conflict. My views as a concerned family member will inevitably be different from those I hold as a human services consultant, regardless of how rationally I approach this subject. I believe, however, that considerable reconciliation of these various positions can be achieved through a systematic assessment of the multiple facets of the managed care issue.

ASKING THE RIGHT QUESTIONS

Key to this assessment is understanding the motivating factors underlying the managed care movement, identifying with precision the specific desired objectives and outcomes, and selecting appropriate methods for achieving the established goals. Once the motivating factors and desired outcomes have been identified, the next step is to assess whether outcomes are compatible with each other. In those instances in which potential conflict exists, it is important to examine alternative strategies for achieving outcomes. Some strategies may heighten the conflict while others may reduce the likelihood that the achievement of one goal will contribute to one's inability to achieve another goal. For instance, most managed care initiatives claim to be directed at reducing the cost of services while protecting against compromising the quality of service. If the strategies for reducing costs do not take into account the impact on access to needed services, the quality will probably be compromised. Conversely, if the methods for achieving quality ignore cost impact, the initiative will almost certainly not succeed in accomplishing this objective.

On the other hand, if potential interventions are assessed in relation to all objectives, the likelihood of overall success is greater. The following example illustrates how one large service delivery system attempted to establish a utilization management system that would be responsive to the multiple objectives of cost, appropriateness, and quality.

ARTICULATING THE CHALLENGE

In Chapter 9 we described the development of a statewide comprehensive services system for children with emotional and behavioral problems and their families. This system, authorized under legislation known as the Comprehensive Services Act for At Risk Youth and Their Families (CSA), represented a radical shift from the way in which services were traditionally delivered. Programmatically, the CSA promoted development of individualized service plans that were family centered as well as community based. Family participation was emphasized, and the use of community support and services was encouraged. In an effort to eliminate fragmentation and disincentives typically associated with centralized, agency-based management of service delivery, the CSA pooled all available funds and allocated these resources to localities for management and distribution. Each locality was required to develop family-focused service planning and communitywide policy and management teams responsible for implementation of an integrated, community-based service system for children and families. Responsibility and authority for management of fiscal resources and services were delegated to local government. While children had to meet several general criteria to be eligible for CSA services, funding was designated for individual children and families and communities were given considerable latitude to develop innovative individualized service plans that were responsive to child and family needs and strengths.

The CSA's first few years of operation were marked by several notable achievements. Some localities restructured their child services delivery system to produce genuinely collaborative working relationships among providers and families. These new organizational entities were able to use their ingenuity and flexible funding to create community-based alternatives for youngsters who previously would have been sent outside the community to receive needed services. Not surprisingly, however, actualization of such a large and complex program required considerable effort by individuals at all levels, and implementation did not always proceed as smoothly or rapidly as originally anticipated. Toward the end of the third year of operation, the executive and legislative branches of state government, as well as many local government entities, began expressing considerable concern about the performance of the CSA service delivery system. Specifically, the overall cost of the program had increased by nearly 20 percent a year. At the same time, many children continued to be placed in expensive, out-of-community residential treatment facilities.

The state's executive council, which was comprised of the heads of the state child-serving agencies as well as representatives of other critical stakeholder groups including parents and providers, recognized the need to take constructive action to deal with these problems. The council's first task was to define the parameters of the problem and identify appropriate remedies. Knowing the generally negative public perception toward strategies designed to control costs in other health and human services sectors, the council wanted to ensure that any changes it might introduce would be compatible with the overall philosophy and principles of the CSA. Thus, any effort to contain costs would have to take place within the context of the CSA's individualized and family-centered service planning and delivery emphasis as well as its focus on maintaining authority and responsibility at the local level. The council considered a number of approaches for dealing with this issue. Some were rejected as insufficient; others were not selected because of the strong likelihood of yielding unintended consequences such as stripping local governments of their appropriate authority and roles as defined within the CSA-enabling legislation. Finally, the council decided to explore the possibility of incorporating concepts and tools of utilization management strategy into the CSA.

"Utilization management" is a broad term that encompasses a wide range of activities intended to improve service efficiency and effectiveness through implementation of a system of rational management strategies. These interventions range from enhancing the quality of information upon which service planning and resource allocation decisions are made to establishing external controls designed to limit access to service. The council was careful to limit its definition of utilization management to those approaches that would provide improved guidance and data to localities without compromising their ability to actually make decisions about which services a particular child and family should receive.

Having selected a general approach, the council decided to hire a university-based research and technical assistance institute to conduct a study to assess the feasibility of incorporating utilization management principles and practices into the CSA delivery system. In response to the council's request that the study address dimensions of quality as well as efficiency within the context of the CSA philosophy and principles stated above, the institute designed a broad-based assessment that would examine an array of factors that might be contributing to performance problems and that would be sensitive to the council's desire to enhance the ability of localities to function in an empowered manner. The study incorporated both quantitative and qualitative methodologies and relied heavily upon input from various CSA stakeholders including consumers, children, and families; local government officials; and service providers. While all parties agreed that sufficient time and resources were lacking to evaluate the outcomes produced by the CSA service delivery system, both the council and the institute agreed that the study should address the question of how the CSA was functioning after three years of operation and that it should test the feasibility of applying utilization management principles to the service delivery system. The institute proposed to assess functioning of the CSA in the following six areas:

1. The knowledge, attitudes, and orientation of state and local staff and administrators regarding service delivery requirements and funding under the CSA.
2. The availability or lack thereof of service resources for localities.
3. The availability or lack thereof of fiscal incentives in the CSA financial system toward cost containment, including whether or not local CSA pool savings should be used for program development.
4. The local ability to develop the necessary clinical assessment of children's strengths and needs in relationship to the appropriateness of their out-of-community placement, including focusing on expected outcome probabilities and monitoring service delivery in relationship to expected outcomes.
5. The overall impact of demographic patterns and service demands on CSA cost and service utilization.
6. Localities where costs have stayed the same or decreased should be considered in the effort, as well as localities where costs have increased significantly.

In regard to the question of feasibility, the institute was asked to assess whether the application of utilization management principles to the CSA would enable the council to improve the quality and efficiency of services purchased in the following areas:

- Reduction in historical cost increase for funded services.
- Reduction in out-of-home placements.
- Reduction in inpatient and residential treatment and length of stay.
- Reduction in recidivism.
- Improvement in youth functioning at home and school.
- Improvement in youth and family satisfaction.

In addition to presenting the findings and conclusions, the institute also was expected to provide a series of recommendations describing what actions would be required to implement a utilization management system that retained the locus of decision making as close as possible to the youth and family for whom services were to be delivered.

CREATING A RECEPTIVE CLIMATE

Everyone involved in the feasibility study process—council members and staff of the institute—recognized what a formidable challenge they were undertaking. The technical requirements of the utilization management system for a large comprehensive program were, by themselves, a daunting task. Added to that was the awesome challenge of gaining acceptance and achieving consensus among a varied group of stakeholders including consumers, providers, and administrators. Finally, the prospect of successfully implementing this enormous project in such a short period of time—the study had to be conducted, analyzed, and reported within four months— elicited considerable anxiety among the participants.

A steering group was formed to guide implementation of the study. The steering group, comprised of institute and CSA staff as well as representatives of stakeholders such as local government and providers, addressed a number of critical implementation issues. Its first task was to define the type of utilization management system to be used in the feasibility test component of the study. In keeping with the council's guiding principle of decision-making authority at the local level, the steering committee opted to pilot-test a decision-support process as the cornerstone of the CSA feasibility study, using the following definition: "The decision-support process provides pertinent information and guidance for individuals and organizations interested in designing, implementing, monitoring, and evaluating services on dimensions of appropriateness, quality, and cost-effectiveness."

The steering committee viewed this form of utilization management as having several advantages. In addition to providing decision makers with a rational, data-driven framework to enhance the quality of decisions, this approach also allowed localities to tailor the decision-making process to the unique conditions of their communities. As defined by the steering committee, the decision-support process would be comprehensive enough to address a broad range of utilization concerns, that is, appropriateness, quality, and cost-effectiveness. Finally, this process would have multiple applications ranging from developing a specific service plan for an individual to designing a comprehensive system of care.

For use in the feasibility study, the steering committee selected the Childhood Severity of Behavioral and Emotional Disorders (CSBED) rating scale, a modified version of a needs-based assessment tool originally developed by John Lyons of Northwestern University. This assessment instrument was designed specifically as a utilization management tool to help decision makers select the appropriate level of care for children with emotional and behavioral disorders. The instrument assesses behaviors according to five dimensions: symptoms; risk factors such as harm to self or others; level of functioning in various settings; comorbid problems such as illness and substance abuse; and system factors, including readiness of the caregiver and community to provide services for a child and family. While the CSBED has a defined, uniform rating scale, localities can establish their own guidelines and criteria for matching child needs with appropriate levels of care. The process is not formula driven as it allows for the introduction of mitigating circumstances that may guide service planning decisions.

The CSBED was used for several purposes in the CSA feasibility study. Individual child profiles of the dimensions of symptom, risk, function, comorbidity, and system factors were generated. These profiles provided descriptions of the children being served at the individual and aggregate levels. A set of guidelines based on symptoms, risk, and caregiver characteristics was defined to compare actual placement levels of children being served by the CSA with level of care that might be expected according to the CSBED model.

The steering committee next addressed the question of how to persuade localities to participate in the feasibility study. Not wanting to increase the work burden of localities or impose yet another state-mandated requirement, the council had been reluctant to require localities to participate. The steering committee decided to offer an invitation to a representative group of localities. In order to reduce suspicion that data from the study might be used in a punitive fashion, localities were promised their identities would not be revealed and that data would be reported in a statewide, aggregate format. As an additional incentive, participating localities would receive a summary of data for their community that would not be made available to anyone else. In order to reduce the burden on localities, all scheduling was done at the convenience of local participants. Interviewers and focus group leaders were instructed to be sensitive to the needs of participants, and a high priority was placed on "customer satisfaction." Arrangements were made to provide refreshments for those who participated in focus groups, and parents and children were given coupons to fast-food restaurants upon completion of the written surveys. Finally, researchers spent time with each participant to explain the rationale and purpose of this study.

Twelve localities, including urban, suburban, and rural counties, agreed to participate. Clinical profiles were developed through an interview process with case managers using the CSBED. Focus groups were held with direct line as well as administrative and policy personnel, and child and parent satisfaction data were collected through a mail survey. In addition to the in-depth assessment of the twelve localities, several methods were used to collect information on a statewide basis. Additional focus groups were conducted with key stakeholders, and brief written surveys were distributed to local CSA personnel, parents, and providers. Child-specific and communitywide demographic data were analyzed in relation to service utilization and cost data for each locality to determine whether specific factors accounted for service pattern and spending and cost differences.

This multimethod approach of assessment was selected for two reasons. First, the designers of the study believed that a complex service system, such as the CSA, could only be understood by looking at a wide range of information sources as well as multiple perspectives. The second reason for selecting this approach had as much to do with ensuring positive outcome as it did with scientific integrity. The designers hoped that by providing stakeholders with information on the purpose and functions of utilization management and offering them an opportunity to provide input into the design of this system, their anxiety might be reduced and receptivity to utilization management strategies might be enhanced.

Following implementation of the study—which was accomplished in a compressed time period of five weeks—the data were collated, entered, and analyzed. The research team then met to consider what conclusions could be drawn from the data as well as what recommendations should be made in response to the application of utilization management principles to the CSA. The group's deliberations were guided by two general principles: First, the conclusions and subsequent recommendations had to be supported by the study's data, and second, the success of any suggested course of action would be dependent upon its ability to address the dual concerns of being programmatically sound and fiscally viable. The research team quickly discovered that achieving this balance was not an easy task. For example, a strategy that relies heavily upon data-driven decision making requires technological sophistication in terms of data collection and analysis as well as decision-maker competence. In addition to requiring substantial investment of resources for training and creative technological capacity, empirically based systems function most effectively when a uniform database is capable of producing coherent reports that can be used at both the local and state levels. The problem with this approach is that any effort to require uniformity would be perceived by localities as directly challenging their ability to tailor the utilization management process to the unique conditions of their communities. Conversely, allowing localities to have complete freedom of choice precludes the possibility of comparing or aggregating locality-specific data. This not only hampers statewide policy analysis efforts; it also limits the ability of localities to learn from each other.

In assessing the potential merits and liabilities of various recommended approaches, the research team considered how each strategy addressed the complex and often competing concerns of the various stakeholders. Besides the uniformity of procedures versus local choice dimension described above, the team took into account whether proposed strategies were responsive to fears that the CSA might be reduced to a service system driven primarily by a bottom-line mentality, and it attempted to achieve a reasonable balance in relationship to the scope of recommendations proposed. Team members wished to avoid the risks at either end of this continuum of offering one or two strategies that might be too limited to effectively address the problems or providing an overly ambitious agenda that might be viewed as impractical and unachievable.

The final report acknowledged that the CSA was achieving many of its primary service objectives, but it also pointed out several areas that were in need of improvement. Researchers concluded that the application of utilization management principles to the CSA was feasible and would, in fact, be welcomed by most stakeholders. While much of the report focused on how to develop and implement utilization management tools, equal emphasis was given to the importance of enhancing localities' ability to collaboratively develop and provide a community-based system of care that was comprehensive and family centered. This conclusion was based on the premise that good assessment instruments are of limited use if providers lack sufficient resources to offer services appropriate to the identified needs of the child and family.

Based on these conclusions, a set of recommendations was offered. In keeping with the thrust of the study, the first recommendation was to develop a comprehensive system of utilization management processes consistent with the CSA principles. In order to address the issue of local empowerment while, at the same time, acknowledging the wide variation and sophistication among political subdivisions within the state, it was proposed that localities be required to operate a utilization management system and that the state provide assistance directly or by contract for gathering, analyzing, and distributing relevant data as well as decision-support guidelines. Wanting to give the state executive council leeway in choosing how to proceed, the authors of the report provided two implementation options: (1) all localities would be required to participate in a single state-supported utilization management system and (2) localities would be given a choice of choosing among a number of state-approved options.

Other recommendations included establishing and realigning fiscal incentives to encourage localities to develop an array of community-based services and offering training and technical assistance to improve localities' capability to develop, manage, and evaluate responsive service systems for children and families. Finally, an initial implementation plan was offered for developing a decision support system and enhancing localities' capacities to provide community-based systems of care.

These recommendations were intended to provide localities with resources and tools that would enhance their abilities to provide services that matched the needs and strengths of at risk youth and families. The recommendations pertaining to decision support processes were designed to help local decision makers' understand what services children and families needed. The other recommendations, including those dealing with realignment of fiscal incentives, strengthening local service capacity, and improving the service contracting process, were intended to assist localities in better understanding how to obtain needed services. While the major focus of these recommendations was to improve the appropriateness and quality of services, it was assumed that the concern about escalating costs would be addressed by reducing use of expensive, out-of-community residential treatment for those children who could be better served in a community-based system of care.

A draft report was distributed to the steering committee as well as to study participants. Based on comments from these initial reviewers, modifications were made to the report to improve its accuracy and readability. The report was next presented to the state executive council. After a thorough review of the report, the council provided a strong positive endorsement of its findings and recommendations. It then charged the institute and steering committee with developing a plan for implementing a decision support process as well as other utilization management strategies. Those of us who had been intimately involved since the inception of the project were surprised and impressed at how well everything was proceeding.

TOO GOOD TO BE TRUE

Participants in large-scale system reform initiatives quickly learn that events do not typically unfold in a simple, linear pattern. Almost always, many individuals and organizations have a vested interest in the outcome of these initiatives. Although these interested parties may have a genuine desire to improve the system that is the focus of attention, these altruistic inclinations are often tempered by their pursuit of more self-serving objectives. The dynamic interplay among various parties working to ensure that individual objectives—as well as system-reform goals—are achieved often sidetracks the process, extending the time required for resolution and producing unanticipated results.

The CSA utilization management initiative was no exception. The final report was distributed to all 140 CSA localities as well as to other interested organizations, including service providers, parent advocacy groups, state agencies, and legislative staff. Judging by the few formal responses the steering committee received, one might have assumed readers either lacked interest or had a high degree of acceptance of the report's recommendations. As the steering committee learned later, neither was the case. Interested parties began to mobilize their resources immediately. Some acted through political channels, expressing their views directly to legislators. Others used formal and informal communication processes to interpret the report and its implications for constituencies. Still others worked within established channels, contributing ideas and suggestions consistent with the vested interests of their constituents.

Because many of these external parallel activities took place outside the view of those managing the initiative and, therefore, remained invisible, several endeavors were quite apparent. Two of the more notable efforts to influence the process were a legislative mandate to incorporate utilization management practices into CSA and an attempt by child-caring agencies to ensure that the utilization management process accommodated their unique interests and requirements.

About the same time the final report of the feasibility study was being written, the general assembly passed a resolution requiring the state executive council to institute a utilization management process for the CSA. The resolution, which carried with it the clout of a legal mandate, stated that all localities that requested supplemental funds, if their regular allocations proved to be insufficient, would be required to institute some form of utilization management. The legislature was clear in its intent not to force localities to choose a particular system of utilization management, but the freedom of choice was qualified by the requirement that the state could develop a set of criteria for utilization management with which each locality would have to comply. The utilization management legislation also directed the state department of medical assistance to make available its utilization review organization to assist in this effort. Attached to the legislation was a budget appropriation of $175,000 for the next fiscal year.

The legislature's action impacted the state executive council process in several ways. First, giving localities a choice to participate in the utilization management process—albeit a choice with some consequence—and stipulating that localities could choose their own particular utilization management systems effectively eliminated the possibility of having a uniform and consistent system. Obviously, the intent of the legislation was to ensure that the prerogative of local choice was preserved. What is not known is whether the legislature's actions were motivated by political philosophy or more mundane forces, such as lobbying groups intent on thwarting further intrusion by the state executive council into the affairs of localities. Whatever the underlying motivation was for introducing this legislative mandate, the impact was clear. Localities would be able to choose whether they participated in the utilization management process; those who opted to participate would have considerable latitude in selecting the method for implementing a utilization management process; and CSA administrators would be faced with a difficult challenge as they attempted to figure out how to provide assistance and support for a diverse and complex array of utilization management approaches.

The designation of the Department of Medical Assistance and its utilization review organization as participants in the utilization management process resulted in a second unanticipated impact. Having two additional parties involved added complexity to the planning process. More important, the Department of Medical Assistance and its review organization were perceived as representing the "medical model." Historically, the interaction among the multiple child-caring constituencies had been characterized by tension concerning this issue. Because all agencies were considered to be equal partners in the supposedly holistic approach, each agency constituency was sensitive about any aspect of the program that might be considered discipline specific. One of the main sources of contention was that mental health agencies were using diagnostic and treatment language and tools that were medically oriented and did not take into account the educational, social, and juvenile justice aspects of children's functioning. Introducing an organization that was directly identified with the medical model rekindled these concerns.

Concern about agency territoriality was manifested in at least two other ways. Representatives from local and state education departments were adamant that one size could not fit all. They argued that the federal Individuals with Disabilities Education Act (IDEA) stipulated that all special education placement decisions had to be determined through the individualized educational planning process (IEP) and established clear boundaries for what constituted acceptable input for the decision process. They stated that the generic utilization management process would be inappropriate for special education since it might dictate actions for the education department that were outside their legal mandate. Advocates for this position also expressed concern about the potential for increasing litigation among parents who perceived that the decision support assessment process might generate recommendations for a service that were in direct conflict with special education requirements.

For a while it appeared that the controversy over inclusion of special education in the CSA utilization management process would undermine the overall effort to introduce a rational planning process into the CSA system. Fortunately, a representative from the state education department who had a strong investment in the CSA's family-centered, integrated system approach, and who understood special educators perceived and actual constraints in regard to this issue, took constructive action. Working with the steering committee, she convened a meeting of local special education officials, CSA representatives, and individuals involved in planning the utilization management strategy. By narrowing the focus of attention to those issues that had a genuine legal basis, the group was able to develop alternative processes that would provide special educators with the assurances they needed while maintaining the overall integrity of the CSA utilization management process.

The second turf issue revolved around the selection of a specific assessment instrument to be used by localities in order to match the needs of each child with an appropriate array of services and level of care. Although each locality had the option of choosing its own assessment method, the state executive council concluded that it would identify one particular assessment tool that would be supported by the utilization management technical assistance initiative mandated by the legislature. Initially, the steering committee recommended use of the CSBED, the instrument that had been used during the feasibility study. Not only had this instrument been specifically designed for utilization management purposes, but it also proved to be relatively easy to administer and produced data that localities found useful. Toward the end of the design phase, a representative from the state department of mental health raised a concern about this use of the CSBED. Several reasons were presented in challenging the appropriateness of the CSBED, but the principal objection was that many localities were already using another instrument that could be used for this purpose. The department's representative argued that introducing a second instrument not only would be inefficient but also would create animosity among local agency personnel who would resent the additional burden of having to use two assessment instruments.

On the surface this proposal seemed reasonable. If another instrument were already in use, it did not make sense to add a second assessment tool. Some members of the steering committee objected, however, to the timing of this proposal as well as the appropriateness of the suggested instrument for utilization management purposes. These individuals felt that the objection was raised primarily to give the state and local mental health agencies, which were the primary users of this instrument, more control over the assessment process. They were concerned that placing mental health agencies in a dominant position would undermine the interdisciplinary focus of the CSA and wondered why the suggestion had been made so late in the design process. They also questioned whether the proposed instrument, which had been designed principally for the purpose of assessing functioning of a child and had been used extensively as an outcome measure, would produce specific information needed to make decisions about the appropriate level of care required to meet children's needs.

This conflict, which shared common characteristics with the dynamic of sibling rivalry, threatened to sidetrack the progress of the steering committee. Some participants feared that if the dissension continued unabated, it was likely that the entire utilization management initiative might be compromised or even destroyed. Recognizing little chance that the conflicting parties would reach resolution on their own, the leadership of the steering committee proposed an innovative method for arbitrating the conflicting approaches.

The identified proponents of the two instruments were charged with convening a group of local representatives familiar with practical aspects of identifying appropriate services for children to participate in a time-limited planning process. The group of local representatives were given the opportunity to review the most recent decision support guidelines as well as the department of mental health's assessment instrument. The group was asked to define characteristics of children who corresponded to various levels of service need as well as to determine whether the assessment instrument could provide specific criteria to define service need characteristics operationally. By turning to a representative group of local CSA stakeholders, the steering committee was able to defuse the conflict as well as to develop guidelines that had been endorsed by future users of the decision support process.

With completion of the guidelines, the next step was to educate CSA stakeholders at all levels regarding the purpose of introducing utilization management approaches and the mechanics of how they would be implemented. Borrowing from management theory, the steering committee decided to begin its orientation with local government officials who had ultimate responsibility for the management of the CSA. A series of orientation meetings were scheduled throughout the state. These sessions were intended to assist local officials to understand the utilization management process and to allow them an opportunity to think through how they wished to incorporate utilization management into their local CSA system. In addition to giving them knowledge, an important goal of this orientation was to begin to develop a sense of ownership among the local decision makers. A description of various alternatives was presented and local officials were told that they could choose if and how they would participate within the coming months. Assurance was provided that training and technical assistance would be available for localities expressing an interest. The local official orientation was followed by training sessions with the persons who had responsibility for the day-to-day operation of the CSA service delivery system. These individuals, who administered individual and service planning functions, were provided with information about how actual utilization management processes might be implemented, and they received a general orientation.

STAYING ON THE TIGHTROPE

The feasibility study and initial development of a utilization management system for the CSA illustrates the difficulty of achieving balance among the multiple goals and interests of a complex service delivery system. Early in the process it became apparent that many of the CSA's original goals, particularly those directed at the provision of assistance to localities through training and the development of databases that could be used for program evaluation, were not being supported to the extent initially envisioned. The amount of effort required for the start-up process as well as changes in state leadership with the election of a new governor made it difficult to implement these aspects of the CSA system. As a result, localities were not always prepared to adhere to the principle of individualized, family-based planning that resulted in children being served whenever possible in community settings. Naturally, the lack of systematic service planning mechanisms had some negative impact on service development, child placement, and cost.

At the same time, the overall climate of the health and human services delivery environment was changing. Greater attention was being given to controlling costs through a variety of mechanisms, including some fairly crude approaches that simply limited access to services without providing either a rational basis or a viable alternative. The psychological resistance to managed care on the part of those concerned with children combined with their strong conviction that children and families should be given comprehensive services that met their needs, generated among these individuals considerable skepticism about whether utilization management principles could be applied to the CSA. Simply demonstrating the technical benefits of such an approach was not sufficient. It was necessary to involve stakeholders in understanding the economic and political realities of the situation and to elicit their assistance in designing a utilization management approach that would be consistent with CSA values and principles.

Reconciling the apparent conflict between CSA's fundamental commitment to respecting local differences and encouraging local empowerment, and the value of utilizing uniform procedures to enhance decision makers' knowledge base about the CSA, proved to be a formidable task. Most participants in the CSA recognized the value of having useful clinical information that would help match children and families with appropriate services. What they objected to was having this matching process imposed on them in a manner that diminished both the individualized basis of service planning and the localities' abilities to make service planning decisions based on the unique needs of their communities. Most of all, CSA stakeholders were opposed to the state dictating to localities how they should provide services.

By involving users of the system—parents, providers, and local officials—in the design of the system through focus groups, surveys, and actual demonstrations of how utilization management approaches might be used, the CSA leadership was able to reduce some anxiety and resistance. The provision of education and training programs directed at helping individuals to understand how utilization management approaches could be incorporated into a locally driven system also contributed to greater acceptance. Despite these constructive efforts, considerable negative feeling persisted about the introduction of utilization management approaches to the CSA. Some of these sentiments emanated from a basic lack of trust of anything the state proposed; some resistance stemmed from fear that these changes would adversely affect the abilities of localities to provide individually tailored service programs. Still others feared that this initiative represented the first step in moving toward an externally controlled managed care system.

As the CSA prepared to launch its utilization management initiative, it was apparent that many of the same questions and concerns constituents had at the beginning of the feasibility study still existed, though hopefully to a lesser degree. Multiple and often competing interests and goals, perennial fear of intrusion from a higher level of government, and lack of adequate resources all contributed to participants' unease and suspicion about introducing utilization management approaches. At the same time, mounting pressures to contain costs and a general shift toward managed care interventions had accelerated fear that more drastic measures would be imposed. Paradoxically, these threats actually enhanced acceptance of approaches that allowed localities to retain control of the decision-making process. This perverse set of incentives may have contributed to the relatively smooth sailing the CSA utilization management initiative experienced initially. Several localities began their own utilization management processes even before the state program was formally introduced. The fact that localities were offered a wide range of options certainly enhanced participation.

While it is premature to assess the degree of acceptance or effectiveness of the CSA utilization management initiative, it is possible to identify some of the factors that have contributed to the initial progress as well as those factors that need to be dealt with to ensure future success. The following have been the major enhancing factors:

- Giving constituencies of the CSA opportunity for input into the design of utilization management initiatives through focus groups, surveys, and work groups assisted the design of the utilization management system.
- Providing considerable orientation and education helped to demystify the concept of utilization management and reduced anxieties associated with the lack of adequate information and understanding.
- Allowing localities to phase in utilization management activities at their own pace fostered a sense of control and allowed the leadership to learn from the experiences of first-round participants.
- Providing tools and support to localities rather than imposing external requirements and constraints enabled localities to appreciate the substantive purposes of utilization management—such as appropriate matching of services as well as cost containment—rather than to focus their intentions on the dynamics that existed between the levels of government.
- Offering a wide range of options that localities could choose from preempted the argument that the program is not responsive to the unique needs of each community.

- Involving users of the CSA system in those situations in which conflict arose enabled the leadership to defuse tension while gaining valuable input from those directly affected by the service system.

Having successfully designed a utilization management approach, the leadership of the CSA faced a new set of challenges as the initiative moved into its implementation phase. The effectiveness of the utilization management effort will, in part, be dependent upon how it addresses the following issues:

- How can government officials and other leaders at the local level be brought into the process? If these individuals become convinced that utilization management can assist them in improving services and controlling costs, it is more likely that utilization management strategies will be applied consistently within that community.
- Will there be sufficient attention given to the training and preparation of persons at the local level responsible for conducting assessment, utilization review, and other components of the utilization management initiative? This task is complicated by the fact that localities are able to choose among several options.
- How can realistic expectations be established and communicated to the multiple stakeholders of the CSA, including legislators? The overall cost of CSA services may be influenced by many factors, including the number of children and families referred for services and the impact of competition on providers' service fees as well as efficiencies achieved through effective management of service utilization. While utilization management strategies can reduce service costs, it is important not to oversell the financial benefit that will accrue from this initiative. Even if the application of utilization management principles reduces cost per child, there is no guarantee that other forces, such as inflation and increased demand for services—that is, an increase in the number of children served—will not offset these financial savings.
- Will the provision of assistance in developing community service capacity keep pace with the progress in assessment technology? Knowing what services a child needs is useful only if those services are available and accessible. Measures should be taken to ensure that local participants do not believe that assessment and utilization review procedures are viewed as panaceas.

Throughout its brief history the Comprehensive Services Act for At Risk Youth and Families has managed to respond successfully to a series of complex and sometimes daunting challenges. By responding in a balanced manner to the programmatic, fiscal, and political forces operating at the local and state levels, the CSA has successfully endured the threats of its formative years and has evolved into a viable though still fragile system of care. As the CSA enters its third generation of executive leadership at the state level—a formidable challenge in its own right—this ambitious reform initiative will need to muster considerable leadership and creativity to put in place a rationally based assessment and planning system that will control costs while also ensuring that children and families receive appropriately responsive services. Whether the proposed utilization management strategy will be sufficient to meet this challenge depends not only on the quality of the interventions and the skill of the leadership but also on the way in which broader societal forces shape policy and practice during the next few years.

POINTS TO PONDER

1. By providing a system that allowed local flexibility, the Comprehensive Services Act gained acceptance from localities but sacrificed uniformity and consistency in procedures and information that could be used to assess the impact of the service system. What are the advantages and disadvantages of an approach that allows considerable flexibility at the local level?

2. The goals of the Comprehensive Services Act were bold and ambitious. Given the magnitude of this proposed reform of child and family services, how realistic is it to expect that the system would be implemented as designed? Discuss possible strategies for transforming Comprehensive Services Act legislation into a viable service delivery system.

3. In recent years the concept of accountability has received increasing attention within the field of human services. The Comprehensive Services Act's initiative to apply utilization management principles to its service delivery system was intended to enhance accountability in relationship to service appropriateness, quality, and cost. What are some of the approaches to promoting accountability in service systems that focus on both service quality and cost containment? What are the advantages and disadvantages of these various approaches?

4. The leadership of the Comprehensive Services Act wanted to avoid the pitfalls of many managed care initiatives. Do you think they succeeded? In what ways is the Comprehensive Services Act utilization management initiative similar to, or different from, other care management efforts? What other strategies, if any, could have accomplished the same goals more effectively?

5. The utilization management feasibility study concluded that the absence of appropriate incentives was, in part, responsible for the Comprehensive Services Act not fully achieving its stated goals. The use of incentives can be a powerful tool for creating change. What are some incentives that might be incorporated into a service system to ensure that services are appropriate, high-quality, and cost efficient?

CLASSROOM TO COMMUNITY

Applying the Concepts of Change

- Creating change is difficult; being on the receiving end is not easy either. One of the significant sources of resistance to change is the anxiety individuals experience when they know that their roles and functions will be different as a result of organizational or system changes but are uncertain about precisely what their new roles will be and how they will be affected. Identify an organization or service delivery system that is currently or will soon be undergoing major changes and speak to several persons who will be affected by these changes. Gather their perceptions of what is happening and how it will impact them. Select persons involved in different aspects of the organization/system, such as direct service provider, administrator, consumer. What appear to be the most salient issues for each? What are the similarities and differences in their perceptions? What are they doing to cope with these changes?

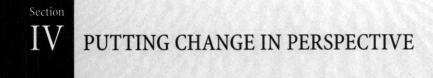

PUTTING CHANGE IN PERSPECTIVE

CHAPTER 11

International Perspective

JOURNEY TO A ONCE FORBIDDEN LAND

HELPING ESTONIA BRING ABANDONED CHILDREN HOME

> *Truly, my brother, if you only knew a people's need and land and*
> *sky and neighbour, you could surely divine the law of its overcom-*
> *ings, and why it is upon this ladder that it mounts towards its hope.*
>
> ~ Friedrich Nietzsche, Philosopher

Working across cultural and linguistic barriers adds to the complexity of human services. This chapter describes the experience of traveling as an American consultant to work with service providers who are starting a new program for children and families in Estonia, a former Soviet bloc country. Despite the differences between the systems and the languages, many of the issues that arise are familiar, with political and personal alliances and conflicts affecting the work of individuals. In addition, the providers described in this chapter are working in a climate of poverty in a newly independent country. The implications of designing and implementing a program that will meet the needs of its target population are evident. This chapter demonstrates the importance of communication, compromise, and sometimes mediation.

~

March 5, 1993—Tomorrow I am scheduled to fly to Tallinn, Estonia, to work with a pediatrician and a small group of individuals he has recruited who are starting an innovative family-focused program. They are attempting to return abandoned institutionalized children to their biological parents or another suitable home. Driving to work, I hear on National Public Radio that this is the fortieth anniversary of the death of Stalin.

I grew up with an image of Russia that never got past the fear of Stalin. We whispered nervously in the dark halls of our elementary school about how, any day, Stalin and the Russian army might invade the shores of the United States. Crouched under our desks during air-raid drills, playing with our dog tags, we fantasized about the destruction created by the hydrogen bomb and wondered who would push the button first. We knew nothing about Estonia or Leningrad. We only knew that Stalin was a very bad guy and that the Russians were our enemies.

Tomorrow I fly to Estonia, a small country given to the Germans in a secret pact just before World War II, ending twenty years of independence, the only freedom Estonians have known during the previous 500 years.

That is, until 2,000,000 citizens of the Baltic states formed a 600-kilometer human chain from Estonia to Lithuania and faced down the crumbling Russian Soviet Federated Socialist Republic.

March 6, 1993—My wife, Nancy, and my sons continue to be enthusiastic and supportive of my trip. I have my moments of doubt. What does a displaced New Yorker who has difficulty understanding the culture of Richmond, Virginia, know about the culture of Estonia? On second thought, Virginia might be a damned good training ground.

Barbara, a nurse at the treatment center, and I have been asked by the Christian Children's Fund, which along with the European Economic Community is cosponsoring the project in Estonia, to work with the project staff to help parents reintegrate these institutionalized children into their homes and to assist the project director in developing organizational strategies for achieving the goals of the project. We have been invited as a follow-up to work done by Suzanne, a school of nursing faculty member from the treatment center, who spent two weeks working with the Estonian project. Barbara will be focusing on parent education, and I will be concentrating on the program development and community networking aspects of the program. Our flight will be long but, hopefully, uneventful. We are both anxious to get started.

March 7, 1993—We land in Helsinki, which is still under a thick cover of clouds after a fresh snowfall. I have never been in Helsinki. Barbara has never been outside of the United States, except for a visit to Canada. We are impressed by Helsinki Airport. It is so bright and clean. My ignorance about Estonia makes me wonder if it will be dreary.

The Estonian Airways jet that we have taken from Helsinki to Tallinn—an old Russian Aeroflot plane—breaks through the clouds and lands at the Tallinn airport under sunny skies. I hope this is a good omen.

We are greeted by Alexander, the senior physician in charge of the project, and Dr. T, also a pediatrician, who is president of the Estonia Central Union for Child Welfare, the agency that initiated the project. Dr. T is cordial, but he takes his leave quickly. Alexander is warm and open, as Suzanne said he would be. Our first surprise comes when we are told that we will be staying in different houses. Barbara will stay at Tervis Sanitorium, which is now the facility used to train parents to work with their children who have asthma and other serious respiratory diseases. I will be staying by myself in a small house next to a medical center about a half mile from the sanitorium.

We meet Ulvi, the project coordinator, and we have a lunch of potato soup, potatoes, pork, and cole slaw. I have not eaten such heavy food in years. We are then told that we will be meeting with the interpreter at the Hotel Viru in an hour—and that we will be eating again.

Our trip to the hotel gives us another perspective on the economic situation in Estonia. After we park the cars, Ulvi goes around to the front of the car, removes her windshield wipers, and locks them in the car. When I ask why she has done this, she confirms my suspicion that it is to protect them from theft. I have seen the same response in New York City, but there the concern is for the security of radio and tape players, not windshield wipers. I wonder if this is an indication of the level of desperation and poverty.

We waste no time getting down to business. The conversation turns quickly to what we are going to present to the staff. In true consulting fashion, we turn the question around and tell them we need to know what they need before we decide what we will provide. Alexander, Ulvi, and the interpreter Neve smile. They say they are getting used to the American way of consulting. To our relief, they also say they like this style.

The conversation is intense and I become caught up in the process of communicating with the Estonians. Although Alexander and Ulvi understand and speak English, using Neve helps considerably. She has an incredible knack for assimilating and translating our long-winded responses, and we quickly reach agreement on a game plan. We will meet with staff as early as possible and ask them what they feel they need to successfully implement the project. We will deal with parent training, community relations, organizational development, and team building. All of the cultural barriers seem to dissolve as we quickly become caught up in the project.

After we identify some obvious training needs, such as helping direct care staff to work effectively with families and assisting Alexander and Ulvi in their program development and supervisory roles, we move directly into discussion of the problems they are having in relating to their oversight committee and city government. It soon becomes evident that they are experiencing some of the same petty jealousies and political jockeying that we are too familiar with in the United States. Initially, Alexander presents the problem with the oversight group as stemming from a difference in management style as well as ideological conflict over the value of the program. Upon closer examination, he reveals that some of the members of the oversight committee are upset about the fact that the grant was given to the project at Tervis Center. We discuss strategies for attempting to involve these individuals in taking ownership of the project, to make them partners in the endeavor. Apparently the Tervis project group has begun this by having the committee meet with its team last week. According to the verbal account, the meeting was successful, and we talk about ways of building on that positive experience.

Looking out from the twenty-second floor in this small private dining room, it is easy to forget how much poverty there is in Estonia, except for one thing. While the skyline is nice, as the sun sets and it becomes dark, it is apparent that many of the lights in the tall buildings are not lit. We ask Alexander, and he confirms our suspicion that people cannot afford to use their electricity. Welcome to Estonia.

I am dropped at my small dwelling next to the medical center and I am, once again, struck by how different it is in Estonia. The medical center, which is a nice-looking older structure, is apparently nearly defunct, a victim of Estonia's process of converting to the capitalistic style of the West. Private health insurance has been introduced, and it appears to have picked up our worst features as well as our best. With the advent of insurance, there is no longer any way to pay for public services offered by this reputable medical center. I need to learn more about what is happening here.

Alone in my little house, I have a moment of panic when I cannot open the lock to my room. I start to think about what I will do, but I successfully suppress my anxiety. Eventually the door opens. I unpack my suitcase and get settled.

The reality of the Estonian experience is beginning to hit me. It seems odd that in the course of a few hours, with the aid of an adept translator, we have been able to establish good communication. We have seen clear indications of the cultural differences between Estonia and the United States and are trying our best to be sensitive to these differences. We also have become aware that so much of what we are dealing with is consistent across our cultures: the social politics of human services, the basic concepts of developing a program, and the dilemmas of clinicians and other human services providers trying to assume leadership roles. I think this will be an exciting trip.

March 8, 1993—Our first full day of working together. We begin the morning by presenting an overview of good planning, management, and supervision. Alexander seems sensitive to the fact that he has not had any formal training in these areas and is eager to learn what we know about these subjects. Although he expresses interest in becoming familiar with theories and rules, he and Ulvi seem open to our less academic approach of presenting a few basic concepts, outlining some options, and helping them to figure out how they would like to approach these tasks. We spend more time discussing the problem regarding the relationship of the committee and the city government and attempt to frame the situation as an opportunity for utilizing these groups as outside resources that can help them in their task of establishing a successful program. We move on to the importance of having a plan that has had input from as many participants and stakeholders as possible. We agree to go through the exercise of developing a plan for the project with them and the team in order to illustrate how this process works. Once again I am struck by how applicable many of the basic tenets are that we have used in our program and community development work. We continually ask them if the material is relevant to their culture, and for the most part they respond affirmatively. At one point, we are talking about how to recruit foster parents through the media. They explain that in Estonian culture, the spokesperson in a televised public service announcement should definitely be the director of the program and not a staff member or some other representative.

By the end of the day we seemed to have established a leadership framework that puts Alexander and Ulvi in a cooperative executive committee role, engaging members of the team as participants in various functions such as evaluation and marketing but making clear that the ultimate responsibility for these functions resides with the management team. Although both Alexander and Ulvi express satisfaction with this approach and seem comfortable, it will be interesting to see what happens tomorrow when we begin working with the entire team.

We have been here less than two days, but I feel very involved with Alexandra, Ulvi, and Neve and am not aware of being thousands of miles from home in a place that would have been totally inaccessible to me less than three years ago.

In the afternoon we visit downtown Tallinn. The shops are more sparsely supplied and reasonably priced than ours, but it is clear that very few people in Estonia can afford most of the items. We go into a store that resembles our convenience stores and are impressed by how long the lines are. We observe these crowded conditions in a number of other stores with large crowds of people congregating at the counters. It is not clear whether they are buying or merely looking.

March 9, 1993—We spend the first part of the morning developing goals and objectives for the project plan. I am pleasantly surprised when Ulvi mentions prevention as a possible goal. Maybe community psychology really has come to Estonia. After some discussion, they decide to focus on strengthening families that may be at risk of abandoning their disabled children. It is fascinating to me to see how relevant the basic principles of problem solving and organization are to the Estonian situation. Later in the morning we observe another example when we teach the group how to brainstorm in order to clearly define the roles and responsibilities of each of the persons on the team. They are extremely grateful for being exposed to this simple tool that we in the United States take for granted.

I have the impression that Alexander and Ulvi are beginning to understand the networking and resource-utilization concepts that are so central to our own program development efforts.

Our initial session with the entire team goes fairly well. It is difficult to comprehend that this team of social workers (a field that did not exist in Estonia until recently and that has only a single university training program with two social-work teachers) and homemakers (we haven't yet figured out exactly what they are) contains two physicians, a master's-level psychologist, and six teachers. I am not certain why these individuals have decided to join the project, but I am fairly confident that the tough economy and difficulty in finding a job have had some influence. Another possible explanation, according to Alexander, is that this is the first social program that has been developed in Estonia. Perhaps this novel, altruistic project attracted their interest.

During a discussion with the second translator, Elle, we have our first exposure to the impact of the ethnic conflict between the Estonians and Russians living in this country. Elle speculates that it would be highly unlikely that Estonian couples would be willing to take in abandoned Russian children and is equally skeptical that Russian families would be ready to bring children into their homes because of their own uncertainties about their future living situations. It is tempting to compare this situation with the problem in the United States of finding homes for African-American children who are unable to live with their biological families.

Food at Tervis Center is plentiful, but it is much heavier and greasier than what I am accustomed to eating. We eat in a large room in which only one of six light bulbs is working. In the morning and at night, Barbara and I eat alone and feel somewhat odd about the special service we are given.

In the afternoon we split into two groups. Barbara works with the social workers and homemakers in defining their roles more clearly and identifying specific needs they would like addressed during training. I continue to work with Alexander, Ulvi, and Neve on the plan. They are certainly ambitious. They wish to develop a model for establishing home-based services for disabled children that can be replicated throughout Europe. I will be grateful if we can successfully accomplish the modest goals of this project. They have the energy and willingness to learn, but the short time frame, their inexperience, and the lack of outside support within their country make this a very difficult project.

By the end of the day we have completed our list of objectives:

1. returning at least 35 abandoned children to homelike settings by October 1993
2. obtaining commitments from at least another 35 families to take in children
3. developing a proposal to fund a project to work with families who are at risk of giving up their disabled children

When the entire group reconvenes we discuss relationships among various members of the team. A number of people state emphatically that the social workers and the homemakers should function as peers with neither of the two assuming a supervisory role for the other. Yet, when the duties of the homemaker are discussed, the social workers nod emphatically that it would be appropriate for the homemakers to roll up their sleeves and help the parents while the homemakers say nothing. By the end of the day, Alexander also observes that the first four people to express their opinions about the day's session were all social workers. The social workers claim it was coincidence. I wonder how long it will take them to learn that just because in democracy we say everyone is equal doesn't mean it is so.

Our experience of working with the translator has been fascinating. Estonia does not have the facilities to provide simultaneous translation. Therefore, we will speak for a couple of minutes in English, then listen while the interpreter translates what we have said into Estonian. Because of Neve's enthusiasm, the message she delivers often sounds better to us than what we originally said, even though we do not understand most of what she is saying. Neve's enthusiastic participation and obvious commitment to the project have led us to the conclusion that there is a new role for translators, that of group facilitator. Her description of what we have said is often much longer than the original message. It is obvious to us that she is trying to help Alexander and Ulvi understand how they should approach this task. They seem to be receptive to her advice.

Before dinner, I visit Barbara at her house where the children and mothers who receive training for respiratory problems also stay. Before long a small group of children gathers around us eagerly seeking our attention. Although the children do not speak English and we cannot converse in Estonian, there does not appear to be a communication barrier.

Returning to my quiet cottage at night, I walk along a deserted, snow-covered road and I think about how odd it is that I am in the middle of this newly liberated country, struggling for its economic and political survival after 500 years of domination, and yet, in some ways everything feels so normal to me. I worry about an angry dog coming at me from the dark, but I have the same fear in any new neighborhood in the United States. I miss my family and look forward to seeing them when I return home. Otherwise I am at ease with the people and the place. How different from the frightened fantasies of a young boy growing up in the 1950s.

March 10, 1993—Today goes very smoothly. Ulvi, Alexander, Neve, and I focus on fleshing out the plan for the project. By using such basic planning processes as goals, objectives, strategies, and an action plan, we are able to develop a specific set of target objectives and activities that may allow them to reach their desired outcomes. At the same time, we have ample opportunity to discuss some basic principles of program development and leadership. For instance, at one point Alexander mentions that Ghassan, the Christian Children's Fund coordinator in Geneva, has a strong interest in developing a social-work training program in Tallinn in order to increase the number of available qualified social workers. Alexander suggests that we add the training of social workers to our goals for the project. After some discussion we conclude that it would be a good idea to incorporate Ghassan's interest in human-resource development but to frame it in strategic planning language. Consequently, we add a goal that addresses increasing capacity to serve at risk families and cite development of a social-work training program as an objective. At another point, Ulvi suggests that we add as a strategy strengthening the program's relationship with its oversight committee.

I think they are getting the hang of it.

Barbara spends the day on practical strategies for working with families and children. In their discussion of how to develop an individual plan for each family, it is remarkable that they incorporate the same planning principles we are using upstairs as we design the overall plan for the project. The social workers and homemakers respond very well to Barbara's down-to-earth approach.

All week I have had a subliminal reaction that something about Estonia does not make sense. Today I realize what it is. Although it is clear that the poverty in Estonia is pervasive, the physical appearance of the environment and the people are incongruous with the traditional definition of poverty. The houses and buildings look like any in older middle-class America. The streets are clean and the people are well dressed—though more somber than in many other places. While I do not claim to understand much of what is happening in Estonia, at least some of this disparity in appearance and reality must be associated with the sudden collapse of the Estonian economy when it switched to a nongovernment-run free-enterprise system.

The most fascinating aspect of our experience is, of course, the people, especially those we work with most closely. Alexander is a thirty-year-old energetic, idealistic physician whose Russian origins obviously put him in a somewhat marginal position within Estonian society. In spite of the fact that he is a workaholic who doesn't take very good care of himself—he has suffered from impacted wisdom teeth since we arrived but refuses to see a dentist—he is a very warm person with a great sense of humor. He is extremely appreciative of everything we do with him and seems to want very much to improve his skills as a manager. His wife, a nurse, is in her early twenties, and they have a three-and-a-half-year-old daughter. He seems conflicted about remaining in Estonia. Last year he considered emigrating from Estonia to a country where he could make a better living—his salary doubled when he accepted the position of director of this project, from one hundred to two hundred American dollars per month. He speaks of wanting to spend some time in the United States to increase his knowledge about running social programs and perhaps to earn additional money.

Ulvi is a tall, attractive woman who appears to be in her early thirties. She is very quiet, possibly because she is not confident about her English, but clearly she has a good sense of what needs to be done and how to do it. Her relationship with Alexander is a classic physician–program manager relationship. She is willing and capable of handling all the day-to-day details of the project while gently nudging him to do the things that he needs to do as project director. The staff seem to respect her a great deal, and I think she will be a very capable project coordinator. One interesting aspect of the disparity between economic reality and appearance is how people dress. Ulvi and the direct-care staff are well groomed and wear nice clothes. However, each of them has worn the same outfit every day thus far. Neve is a born capitalist. She has incredible initiative and drive, and her intellectual abilities continue to amaze us. There are times when I think that I could probably leave the room and she would carry on the instruction quite nicely without me. Not only is her English excellent, but she speaks in a way that would make it easy to believe that she comes from Los Angeles or Long Island.

At night we go to an organ concert performed by an eighteen-year-old prodigy from St. Petersburg, Russia. It is held in an old and very attractive church. We have difficulty concentrating on the music since the temperature must be close to freezing and we are required to check our coats before entering the sanctuary. Afterward, Alexander takes us to a nice restaurant where we have a bottle of beer, full dinner, and dessert. The cost for the three of us: the equivalent of thirteen American dollars.

March 11, 1993—Today I discover that some organizational dynamics cut across cultural boundaries. After a successful morning of fleshing out the operational plan for the project, I meet with Alexander to work with him on his expressed need to learn more about being a good manager. The discussion soon becomes focused on some very personal concerns about his ability to lead the project. It is a productive discussion, though somewhat odd to have an interpreter inserted into the middle of an intense communication concerning the psychological vulnerability of the project director. It becomes apparent that Alexander is considerably frustrated about the way in which Ulvi and other members of the team do not respond to his authority. We talk about how he might modify this situation, and we end with an agreement that he will spend some time with Ulvi discussing how they can resolve these conflicts.

Less than five minutes later Alexander receives a phone call about bringing another American consultant over to the project for an extended period of time during the spring. He goes downstairs to mention this to Ulvi and returns feeling quite frustrated that she has taken a position contrary to his on this issue. His interpretation is that she does not want another consultant because of her lack of confidence about her fluency in English. This reaction surprises the interpreter, who does not understand why they might need someone else for such a long time period when they will be busily engaged in working directly with the children and families of the project.

Even in good programs, wherever they may be, lack of good communication and divergence of perception seem to be prevalent.

While some patterns are common across cultures, others are idiosyncratic, and one's own cultural bias makes another culture's norms seem odd. Barbara and I go to dinner with two of the project staff. We eat at a restaurant called the Galaxy, which sits about 600 feet above the city in the structure that holds the city's television tower. As in other establishments, we are required to check our coats before entering the restaurant, whose climate was par for the course by Estonian standards. It is probably in the high 50s or low 60s Fahrenheit. We had been told earlier in the day that this custom was practiced in order to maintain the proper environment in a restaurant. Dining out is a special occasion for Estonians, and the site of someone's coat hanging over a chair would detract from the elegance of the setting.

This restaurant is elegant, at least as measured by 1940s American standards. The glass wall surrounds the circular restaurant, giving one a 360-degree view of the city and its surrounding area. The ceilings are shiny black metallic panels that create an art deco impression, and the waiters wear black pants, white shirts, and black bow ties.

With all of this attention to ambiance, it seems somewhat odd to have cheap American rock 'n roll blaring from the restaurant speakers. To make matters worse, it is not even good rock 'n roll, and apparently they have only one tape, which they play over and over.

I suppose the Estonians would find our habit of keeping our coats when entering a restaurant on a cold winter night to be somewhat gauche.

In this small country with its faltering economy, absence of technology, and fierce spirit of independence, I find myself leading a much simpler life. Back at the sanitorium after dinner, I return to my quiet cottage, being careful not to slip as I walk the ice-covered road. I work on my journal for a little while, wash out my socks, underwear, and shirt in the sink, and read a few pages of my book before falling asleep. There is a television, but I have no desire to watch it. There is a telephone, but it is of no use to me. Other days, I have turned on the radio to catch a few minutes of "Voice of America" or to listen to some music, but that is the extent of my contact with the outside world.

I miss Nancy and the kids and wish they were here to share this experience with me. But I do not really miss the other conveniences and complexities of life in the United States. Perhaps I would if I were to stay longer, but for now my narrow bed in my stark, monklike room is a fine substitute for the large comfortable water bed in our beautiful contemporary home in Virginia. The stimulation and wonder I am finding in my experience with the brave people of this pioneering project in a country that has been free for less than three years is more than enough to keep me satisfied for the time being.

March 12, 1993—Another exercise in community psychology. The plan we are developing calls for staff to solicit public involvement in several ways. They need to recruit parents and foster parents to accept the children returning from the home; they want to attract sponsors to provide funding for family support; and they wish to garner general public acceptance and support in order to persuade the government to assume responsibility for the program after grant funding ends.

In a brainstorming session yesterday, we decided that it might be helpful to create a message that links the "Bringing Abandoned Children Home" project theme with Estonia's newly won independence. At first, we considered a message using concepts of freedom or independence, but after some deliberation Alexander and Ulvi decided that a stronger theme would be to connect the Estonian people's transformation from helpless victims to empowered citizens who have reclaimed their homeland with the plight of the children who have been abandoned and who now are hoping to be returned home. I suggested that one way to accomplish two objectives at the same time would be to invite one or more of the committee members, who have displayed some ambivalence toward the project, to lend their expertise in crafting the message and deciding how to deliver it. This would give the committee members an opportunity to take some ownership of the project and provide the staff with some much needed public-relations consultation. Alexander and Ulvi were excited about this prospect and promised to arrange a meeting.

The vice mayor has agreed to meet with the staff late this afternoon. Alexander, Ulvi, Barbara, and I meet with the staff to explain our objective and to gain their support and involvement. They take to the idea immediately and, through brainstorming, come up with a slogan and some other information that might be included in the message. The slogan is "Eestimaa On Taas Merkodu Toome Ka Lapsed Koju Tagast," which translates roughly to "Estonia is our home again. Let's bring our children back home." They also want to include an English version that Barbara and I have proposed: "We Estonians are no longer victims. We have come home to freedom. Let's also bring our abandoned children home."

It does not take us long to discover that the vice mayor is a man who thinks very highly of himself and is more interested in impressing us with his erudition than in helping with the project. After a few false starts, we are able to focus on the task. The vice mayor states that the message, as written, will not be appropriate for a government body such as the parliament but might be suitable for the general public. He proposes that the staff do some personal marketing research by presenting the message to one person they know each day for the next ten days and asking them if they understand the message and what impact it has on them. This will give them a sample of approximately one hundred people on whom to test the message.

The vice mayor and I have a lengthy discussion about the project, how I view Tallinn (solicited by him), and whether it would be worth exploring the possibility of developing relationships between Tallinn and Richmond. I tell him that I understand that this project is very important to Estonia since it is the first project sponsored by the European Economic Community and they will certainly be scrutinizing it carefully to see whether other larger investments in Estonia should be made in the future. I explain that the staff of the project seem very enthusiastic and competent, but their energy alone will not ensure success. The project will only achieve its objectives if broad-based support is received from the government and other influential groups. He concurs with this opinion and agrees to work with the project to gain support. He even volunteers to include a presentation of the project at an ecumenical conference that will be held in Estonia later this year.

No one leaves convinced that the vice mayor will become an avid supporter, but I think the staff understands that they must work to encourage people in a position of influence to help them become involved and assume some ownership for the project.

The dynamic of a community program trying to solicit support from the city fathers and mothers is a familiar one, but playing it out in a place whose culture and history are so different from ours is both fascinating and challenging. Incidentally, the vice mayor has invited Barbara and me to meet with him on Monday in his office to explore relationships between Tallinn and Richmond. I am looking forward to this discussion.

Katrin, a pediatrician who is also working as a social worker in the project, invites us to come with her to a friend's house for coffee and sandwiches. The couple and their two young children live in an old, fairly rundown flat just outside the center of the city. The apartment is odd shaped, with two kitchens, each of which has an adjoining room. They explain that up until several months ago their apartment consisted of a small kitchen and one room. They had to share a bathroom in the hallway with all of the other tenants of the building. Fortunately, they were able to obtain a second apartment and remove the wall that separated the two. We receive a firsthand view of how difficult it is to live in Estonia. The husband is a businessman who spends all his time running around trying to find opportunities. From what we gather, he is not very successful. The mother, a well-educated woman who had been a physical education teacher, stays home with the children all day and barely sees her husband. In some ways, their situation is very similar to a struggling young couple in the United States trying to raise a family and achieve financial success, or at least stability. At another level, there is no comparison between the challenges, instability, and obstacles that exist in the two countries.

March 13, 1993—My experience in Estonia just keeps getting better. We process yesterday's meeting with the vice mayor with Alexander and all of the other project staff, except Ulvi, who has another appointment. They all state how important it was that the vice mayor, who is an influential person, met with them to discuss how they might organize and deliver their message about the project. They feel that he is interested in the project and will support it. Following their comments, the staff ask our views of what had occurred at the meeting. I begin by stating the positive aspects: the vice mayor had been given an opportunity for input, thus increasing the likelihood that he would take some ownership of the project, and it seemed as if he might make some effort on behalf of the project. I was, however, concerned about what appeared to be a lack of clear communication between the project staff and the vice mayor. I was disturbed by his pompous, self-serving attitude and wondered why they had responded so passively to his nonproductive behavior. It is, of course, a rhetorical question. Seeing the stone-faced people on the streets staring straight ahead as they pass us, speaking with young waiters in restaurants who appear to be afraid to smile, and knowing what we do about the oppression the Estonian people have experienced, it is not difficult to know why the project staff have been so diffident and passive in the presence of the vice mayor. In spite of knowing all of this, I want to ask why they behaved so meekly, if for no other reason than to demonstrate the importance of how they communicate about their project with members of the community, including His Honor, the Vice Mayor of Tallinn.

Yet, even as I ask the question, I feel a twinge of guilt, knowing how easy it is for an outsider to blithely confront them with the importance of being assertive. In the United States we are almost always free to confront authority without worry about consequences. Here, even in the recent past, it has obviously been very different.

My question opens a floodgate of discussion, during which they reveal how it is difficult to break the old habits of responding to authority, how they felt at a loss to know what to say that would not offend him and alienate him from the project. They are pleased that I have emphasized that those outside of Estonia will view the project's success as being dependent upon the support received from the government, and they feel that the vice mayor will listen to this message since it comes from an outsider rather than from one of them.

This interchange leads us to a discussion of communication skills. Barbara and I talk about the value of acting assertively as opposed to responding either passively or aggressively. She explains to them that their project is more likely to be supported if they present it in a positive, enthusiastic manner rather than using a self-effacing, tentative approach. She illustrates this point by asking whether they would be more likely to buy a car from someone who simply said that the automobile was okay and hoped they would be interested in buying it or from someone who expressed pride in the performance of the vehicle and the company that made it. They unanimously express their preference for the latter and tell us they will work on trying to communicate more assertively.

Following this discussion, we launch into a team-building segment. Members of the group, including Alexander, are asked to evaluate the current status of the team in relation to its orientation toward productivity and personal relations. We ask them to evaluate their status from the perspective of management staff as well as that of other members of the teams. Interestingly, their assessment of the two groups' perceptions of the team is fairly close, with both groups falling in the middle to middle-high range of both personal relations and productivity. No one rates the team as very low in either category, and they perceive that management leans a little more toward productivity than the other team members.

They are then asked to present their ideas about how the functioning of the team could be improved. They offer a number of suggestions, ranging from having better working conditions to moving from the training to the action phase so they can begin to recruit families. Their comments are evenly divided between personal relations and productivity-oriented recommendations.

When they are finished, Alexander does a good job of summarizing their comments, offering validation for their concerns and providing information on what management staff are doing to address these concerns. He speaks very clearly and definitively—at least as indicated by his body language and the interpreter's translation, and the group listens attentively.

For the first time, I feel as if Alexander is communicating in a manner consistent with his position as project manager and, even more encouraging, as a potential leader.

While we are engaged in some ice-breaking exercises associated with team building, I learn about an additional complexity in cross-cultural training. We ask everyone to write on a piece of paper three things about themselves that no one else is likely to know but that they would be willing to share. The papers are handed in and redistributed and participants are asked to use their ingenuity to find out who has written the paper they have received. As soon as Barbara gives the instructions, we both realize that we will not understand what is written on the papers we have been given since they are written in Estonian and that our papers will be dead giveaways since they are written in English. We improvise by asking Neve to first translate our three attributes into Estonian and then to translate from Estonian to English the papers we have received.

I continue to be impressed by how appreciative the staff are of our training. They not only thank us for working with them but also want to be certain we express their appreciation to Suzanne for recognizing their need for additional assistance. It makes me realize how much we take for granted in the United States. It also bothers me that many of our human services workers and agencies have so much more in the way of resources and yet make considerably less effort to provide the best possible services they can. Perhaps we can do a staff exchange with Estonia.

We liberate ourselves by promising Alexander that if he lets us out of his sight we will be very careful and not do anything to put us at risk. Katrin drives us downtown, and when she drops us off we feel as if we have been released from a long stay in an institution. We eagerly explore the downtown area and, in spite of the fact that most shops close early on Saturday, we have a good time.

After wandering around in the old city for a few hours, we find a nice-looking restaurant and have another four-course dinner for approximately $6.50 per person.

Although we do not return home for another five days, we only have one more full day of work with the project staff. It is frustrating to think that there is so much more that they need to do before the project can fulfill its purpose, but I feel they have a fairly good foundation. If they remain a cohesive team and are able to figure out how to reach their target audiences—parents, prospective parents, potential sponsors, and the government agencies—they stand a very good chance of succeeding.

March 14, 1993—We spend our first day off from work taking a quick tour of the city with Neve, shopping in the old city, and spending the evening with Alexander's sister and her family in their home outside of Tallinn. The only bad part of the day is that it is foggy and damp, which makes it difficult to take good pictures.

During our two-hour historical tour of Tallinn, Neve shows us some of the new suburbs and a few places that have special significance for Estonians, and she points out some of the highlights in the old city. The most moving site for me is the open-air bowl in Kadriorg Park, where the Tallinn Song Festival is held every five years. Up to 200,000 people watch 30,000 children perform Estonian folk songs. According to Neve, the highlight of the festival is seeing that many young people singing Estonian songs that were not accepted as legitimate by the Russians during the Soviet domination.

The strong sense of nationalism among the Estonians is explained during our tour. With a 500-year of history of domination by other countries, including a particularly oppressive reign by the Soviets during the past fifty years, the Estonians have a very strong desire for an independent identity.

During our trip to Alexander's sister's home, we learn, unfortunately, that this strong sense of nationalism also has negative aspects, some of which have seeped into the Abandoned Children's Project. The children's homes are filled with children of both Estonian and Russian lineage. Alexander explains that the issue of which children will be included was discussed by the project staff. Sentiment was strong that their efforts should be limited to returning Estonian children since this would be compatible with the current national spirit. Alexander, as the only Russian member of the project team, is obviously disappointed and frustrated by the discriminatory attitude toward Russian children. It is not clear to us what the outcome will be, but the mere presence of such an attitude makes me sad and introduces a negative element to an otherwise marvelous project. It must be difficult for Alexander to function in a leadership role, knowing that such pervasive prejudice exists. It's odd to think of the Russian people occupying a position in Estonia similar to that of blacks and Hispanics in the United States.

We have a nice visit with Alexander's sister's family. They live in a spacious house in a rural area, with a collective barn across the street in which they keep a cow, a pig, and several chickens. Alexander's sister is a veterinarian, and her husband is a mechanic. They have three healthy and happy young children between the ages of two and six. The children are very eager to play with us and ask their parents when they can visit our home. In spite of the nice surroundings they live in, I am once again taken aback when I learn that Alexander's sister earns the enormous salary of $40 per month.

As our trip begins to wind down, I am aware of how much I have become involved with the Estonians. In an odd way, this visit has opened up a cultural identification for me for the first time. I have never identified strongly with any national or religious group. I don't remember my mother speaking about any cultural ties, and my father, who was orphaned at age six, did not seem tied to his religious or ethnic heritage. I suppose my feelings about Estonia are not totally surprising, given the fact that my mother's parents were from Hungary and my father's family came from Lithuania, both countries that have experienced considerable oppression at the hands of the Russians—as well as the Germans—during the past half century. I wonder if I will sustain my intense interest in Estonia once I return to the States.

March 15, 1993—Late this afternoon, the other shoe drops.

We leave early in the morning to go to Tartu with Alexander. We spend a few pleasant hours touring Tartu University, walking around the town square, and having lunch at his parents' home. Tartu University, the second-oldest institution of higher education in the former Soviet Republic, is situated on a very attractive campus on a hill overlooking the center of town. It is tempting to make comparisons between Tartu University and the College of William and Mary, which is a mere sixty years younger. The main exception, other than size—Tartu is much smaller—is that Tartu seems to have retained more of its original status than William and Mary: long on tradition and short on creature comforts, like most of the rest of Estonia.

Alexander's mother prepares a large and delicious Russian meal, complete with all the fixings—meat, potatoes, a mixture of sour cream and cottage cheese, and light and dark bread, not to mention beets, carrots, and cabbage.

During this trip we learn that Alexander was somewhat of a child prodigy, having been the junior national chess champion for Estonia, which allowed him to travel throughout the Soviet Republic to compete. Somehow the knowledge of his superior skill in chess does not surprise either Barbara or me. He has an incredibly quick mind, and one has the feeling that he is aware of everything that is going on around him, in contrast to his somewhat timid and self-effacing interpersonal style.

When we return to Tallinn, Alexander drops us off at the vice mayor's office. Apparently, however, we either misunderstood or were not given accurate information previously. The man we thought was the vice mayor actually turns out to be a councillor, or a special advisor to the vice mayor. We wait a while for him as he rushes through his appointments—according to the project staff and our own observations, he is always looking at his watch and seems ready to rush off to his next meeting. When we are finally escorted into his office, along with a friendly young woman who turns out to be the national director of the Special Olympics Project, the councillor quickly gets to the point—which is when the other shoe lands square in the middle of the solar plexus of the Abandoned Children's Project.

The councillor tells us he is concerned about the project and "Mr. K" (Alexander). His primary concern about the project is that the people who signed the original agreement underestimated its difficulty and made a commitment to returning 100 children to their families or foster parents by the end of October 1993. He also explains that Alexander is in a tenuous position since he is being paid to direct this project as well as to be the senior physician at the Tervis Children's Center. He is worried about Alexander's ability to organize and manage the project successfully while carrying out his other duties, and he is disturbed by how Tervis staff are also being used in the Abandoned Children's Project, raising the specter of conflict of interest.

The councillor underscores the importance of this project, which is funded by the Christian Children's Fund and the European Economic Community (EEC), to the future financial well-being of Estonia. He describes in graphic detail how the EEC's army of bureaucrats in Belgium does nothing but look for mistakes that may have been committed by projects under its sponsorship.

As I listen to the councillor, it is unclear whether he is trying to impress us with his knowledge of the politics of the EEC or he wants us to know that we are involved in a losing proposition. Perhaps he simply wants to enlist our assistance. To my relief, he asks whether we think the target goals of the project are realistic and whether we might be able to include in our report to the Christian Children's Fund (CCF) an assessment of what might be achieved in the next seven months. I tell him that Barbara and I concur with his opinion that returning 100 children in this time period is unrealistic, even for a well-established program. I also ensure him that the commitment, skill, and energy level of the staff are as good as anyone can hope for and that we feel they have a viable plan and are ready to begin work. Possibly remembering my admonition in an earlier meeting that outsiders will certainly consider the role of associated government agencies in assessing the project's success or failure, he ensures me that he wants very much for the project to succeed and will do everything he can to support it. I tell him I will communicate our opinion about the project not being able to meet its target of 100 children. I will propose instead that the project can realistically reach the objectives stated in the plan we developed with Alexander and Ulvi: returning thirty-five children by October, obtaining commitments from thirty-five other families to take children, and developing a list of children who might be considered for the program in the future. He seems pleased by this proposal and asks that I send him a copy of the report I send to the CCF.

We spend a few minutes discussing the establishment of an ongoing relationship between Tallinn and Richmond and agree that we will send him a formal letter proposing that we explore this possibility. We leave on a cordial note and go to the post office finally to mail our postcards.

Leaving the meeting I have several reactions. On the one hand, the councillor, while still coming across as somewhat pompous, actually seems more interested in the well-being of the project and seems to be more approachable than in our last meeting. Perhaps the politician in him rises to the occasion of performing for a group.

On the other hand, I am quite worried about what might happen to Alexander and the Tervis Children's Center, not to mention the project. The councillor tells us that later this year the sanitorium will become the property of the city. We already know from Alexander that a number of alternative uses for the property have been discussed, including developing a program for the elderly that will be sponsored, in part, by the Swedish Baptist Church. Alexander's position is clearly tenuous and is not helped by the fact that he is a Russian in the midst of a strong surge of Estonian nationalism. While I feel good that we have given him some good management and leadership skills and tools, I am less confident that he will be able to finesse the political minefields and interpersonal challenges that lie in his path. I also have a much clearer understanding of the vague questions he has asked during the past week about coordinating the use of Tervis resources with the Abandoned Children's Project and his trepidation about not being able to trust city government.

The first thought I have is that we are faced with a classic consultation and technical-assistance dilemma. Who is our client and how should we relate to all the players? After some discussion, Barbara and I agree that we need to let the CCF know about the complexities of the Tallinn situation, as well as the need to reexamine the initial objectives of the Abandoned Children's Project. We also will comply with the councillor's request to copy him on our written report to the CCF. We do not see any need to include all of the details about the dynamics of Tallinn's political organization in our written report.

At the same time, we need to lay out all of the issues and problems for Alexander and Ulvi tomorrow and try to assist them in working out a perspective and, hopefully, a tentative game plan for how to handle this volatile situation. I am worried because, given the transfer of ownership of the property to the city, I believe there is a strong likelihood that the children's respiratory program at Tervis, which probably can be handled on an outpatient basis (though I doubt the city will assume this responsibility), will be shut down. My concern is not so much directed at the closing of the program but at the impact this will have on Alexander and how he will handle trying to ensure that the Tervis property remains a children's facility, even if the specific nature of the program needs to change. I am also concerned about how these dilemmas will impact how Alexander and the staff of the Abandoned Children's Project function.

I plan to speak candidly to Alexander and Ulvi about these matters tomorrow. It will be a very challenging day; even before we talked to the councillor, we had a full agenda with more than we can possibly handle during our last day of work with project staff. Barbara and I agree that we should not raise the issues discussed by the councillor until after Alexander and Ulvi have presented the overall project plan to the staff and the social workers and homemakers have begun to work on filling in their parts of the plan.

Tomorrow will be a difficult day. This would be a tough situation to work through under normal circumstances, but with the language and cultural differences added in, it becomes an even more awesome task. I hope I am up to the challenge.

March 16, 1993—The rain this morning is the first since we've been here, though it has been gray and gloomy for the past four days. It reminds me of upstate New York, with the snow and ice melting into slush and exposing the dirty roads and ugly brown ground. I think I am ready to go home.

In spite of the gloomy weather, we have a smooth and productive day. Alexander and Ulvi accept the news of our meeting with the councillor without much reaction. They explain that they have worked through their problems with this man, are prepared to work with him—though they do not trust him—and are ready to move on. I wonder how much denial is in their rational approach, but I do not see any point in pushing the issue at this time. I would like to believe that our training has given Ulvi and Alexander a better perspective on the political aspects of human services, but I suspect that their calm reaction can be attributed to insight gained from our discussions. In the back of my mind I suspect that the Estonian people, having been oppressed for such a long time, feel a sense of futility when it comes to dealing with political authority figures.

Both Barbara and I are surprised also by how much material we are able to cover during our last day. The social workers and homemakers appear enthusiastic about their ability to develop a program for families and children, and they express appreciation to Barbara for giving them practical knowledge and skills. Alexander and Ulvi have a good discussion about their respective leadership styles and appear to have reached a comfortable balance working together as a management team—at least for the moment. In the afternoon we have a unique experience. We are interviewed by an Estonian radio reporter who will be airing a one-hour program on her show this coming Saturday. The experience is unique because the reporter does not speak English and we have to use Neve to translate her Estonian to English and our English to Estonian. The interview goes well, as far as we can tell, and I am impressed by the sophistication of the woman conducting the interview. She is aware of the significance of the project and is curious to learn about our experience in the States and the issues and problems we anticipate the staff will encounter as the project gets underway.

Apparently the city councillor also arranged for an announcement about the project on another radio station, and the staff are very pleased that he has shown his support in a tangible fashion.

Let the marketing begin!

On our last evening in Tallinn, Alexander arranges for the entire staff to go out to dinner with us. Initially, some anxiety arises because Alexander had mentioned going to a sauna restaurant where people can eat and drink and then partake of a sauna. The anxiety arises because the Estonian custom is for people to shed all their clothing in the sauna and, in this case, the sauna will be coed.

Alexander refuses to confirm or deny whether he is sticking to his original plan, but most people agree to go to dinner, especially since he mentions that the sauna is optional.

To our surprise, the restaurant he chooses is not a sauna but a wonderful little cafe built into the wall that surrounds the old city. It is owned by a potter, and a small shop adjoining the cafe sells the nicest craft work that we have seen anywhere in Estonia. The meal consists of a wide assortment of appetizers accompanied by locally produced wine and beer.

Just as impressive as the atmosphere and food, however, are the staff of the project. They all dress up in their best outfits and are as excited as little children attending their first birthday party. Once again, I am struck by the enthusiasm and energy of the staff, their appreciation of even the smallest events, and the enormous contrast between their ability to draw satisfaction from the little that they have and the blasé attitude of most Americans toward the abundance of resources and stimulation available to them. In some ways, our dinner reminds me of the prom Nancy held for students of the Toyota Family Literacy Program. The people in her program, mostly poor African-American women, participated eagerly in all of the events of the dance, including the crowning of the queen. Their exuberance certainly matched that of the traditional teenage student going to the senior prom.

Our last evening in Estonia is both moving and difficult. I feel very good about the work we have done with the staff. Although we have not had time to prepare them to the extent we would want—that is, for us to feel confident they can go out the next day and run the program smoothly—I believe we have helped them develop a good perspective and have exposed them to the essential skills and tools needed to effectively implement a program to return children from institutions to a homelike setting. My interaction with Alexander, Ulvi, Neve, and the other project staff has developed beyond the conventional consultant–consultee relationship. We also have become good friends. And I consider myself extremely fortunate to have been given the opportunity to work with these courageous, committed people in this fascinating country during such a unique and exciting period of its history.

I am certain that my intense feelings about all of this and the difficulty I am having saying goodbye account for much of the uneasy feeling I am experiencing. I wish it were easier to express these intense feelings more directly. But that is not my nature, and I feel some reticence on the part of the Estonians to have our last evening be anything other than a celebration and a time of happiness. Given the bleak conditions they live in, I can certainly understand and appreciate their desire to focus on the positive aspects of our experience.

But my uneasiness is even more complex than my personal style and the perception of our Estonian hosts' desire to remain upbeat. Even as I try to dictate my thoughts and feelings, a vehicle that is usually cathartic for me, I am having difficulty putting what I feel into words.

I am not certain of this, but I believe that at some level my uneasiness comes from my fear of what will happen to this project. Once again, the comparison between the plight of Estonia and the Abandoned Children's Project seems so apt. After a little more than two years of independence, Estonia is still in such a precarious position, with its economic instability, political uncertainty, and its location at the foot of the great Russian bear, a creature whose history has been filled with violent exploitation and whose own current condition is certainly labile.

Likewise, the courage of the project staff, their willingness to take risks, and their commitment to helping reunite children with families, must be considered in the context of the project's precarious position. Not only is it unclear whether or not there is real support from the government, but the project also seems to be entangled in the political battles of the future use of the Tervis Sanitorium. Alexander is an incredibly bright and dedicated individual, but he has neither the skill nor the support to take on such powerful forces.

I am struck by the obvious parallel between the project and Tervis and our situation at the Virginia Treatment Center for Children. I need to be careful not to project too much of myself into this situation. We are still very much at risk of losing the essential identity of our hospital, though I think we are beyond the point of needing to be concerned about our physical survival. Unfortunately, the same cannot be said of the program in Estonia. And for the staff, whose options are far more limited than those of us in the States, the stakes are considerably higher.

So, even as I bask in the warm afterglow of this exhilarating, once-in-a-life-time experience, I cannot help but feel somewhat uneasy about the future prospects of the program, its staff . . . and the country. And just as my involvement in this experience is so much more intense than in other consulting situations, even good ones, my uneasiness about the future is more than the usual paternal, letting-go reaction of an advisor who becomes involved in a program, offers counsel, and then returns to the safe haven from which he came.

Perhaps time will enable me to sort out these feelings more intelligently and may even take the edge off my anxiety about what will happen in the future. Perhaps time—and circumstances—will even be kind to the project staff and spare them from the harsh realities that threaten their program and their country. These are factors that I cannot control and, therefore, I must learn to accept the uncertainty of what will happen.

Some things, however, I am certain will not change over time. I know that the brief period I spent in Estonia will remain etched forever in my mind as an incredible, uplifting experience, a time of intense engagement, renewed appreciation for how good people can be, and, for me, a lifelong agnostic, as close to a meaningful spiritual experience as I probably ever have achieved. The intellectual challenge of trying to teach Ulvi and Alexander how to be managers and leaders, and the personal satisfaction gleaned from their small successes; the amusement of watching Neve switch from her role as translator to group facilitator as she launched into a passionate monologue that far exceeded my original statement; the joy of seeing the team come up with a practical plan for preparing families to accept the children into their homes; the awe of watching the staff cheerfully and diligently putting together a program in spite of their lack of resources; and the excitement of being part of what the radio reporter called "this missionary effort" in the new Estonia—all of this fills me with a sense of excitement and wonder that I have not felt for a long time and that I will not soon forget.

When I left for Estonia I was in a fairly deep rut. I felt a sense of accomplishment about what we had been able to do at the hospital, as well as how we had been able to pull it back from the brink of extinction. I also felt a strong affection for and attachment to the people with whom I work. But I had never considered the role of hospital director as an integral part of my identity, and the excitement of the job had long since vanished. Whether my funk was due to burnout, absence of a creative challenge, midlife crisis, or some combination of these, I felt trapped and wanted to find a new challenge.

What I found in Estonia is definitely a challenge. I don't know what impact it will have on my personal and professional outlook, and it is too early to know whether it will alter the course of my career activities. I do know, however, that for the moment I feel renewed. I also know that if Alexander or any of the others ask for my help, I shall not hesitate to respond.

POINTS TO PONDER

1. Identify several obstacles faced by the Estonian workers in developing their project. How do these compare to your experience with human services organizations in the United States?

2. One of the primary issues in this chapter is communication. How does the author encourage communication and address the problems that occur when people are not clear or direct with each other?

3. How do you view the role of a consultant?

4. How would you approach the situation with the councillor? How would you approach the tension between Alexander and Ulvi, the two leaders of the project?

5. At the time the Abandoned Children's Project was initiated, Estonia was undergoing dramatic political and social changes. Can you relate any of the forces influencing change described in Chapter 1 to the experience in Estonia? What do you consider to be the major differences between introducing human services innovation in Estonia and in the United States? Are there substantive, stylistic, or contextual differences?

CLASSROOM TO COMMUNITY

Applying the Concepts of Change

• Select a country in which you have an interest. Choose an issue that has particular importance in that country due to contemporary political, economic, or social reasons. First, think of a program that might be most needed at this time. Putting yourself in the role of consultant with experience in the field, design a plan for entering the country and working with the service providers who will design and implement the program. Pay attention to the possible obstacles you might encounter and how you would proceed.

CHAPTER 12

Parents' Perspective by *Jeri Baker*

THE HEROINE'S ODYSSEY

The Child Services System Through the Eyes of Parents

> *She would just talk with him and any time he had a problem, like anger would strike him or anything, she would say, "Pick up the phone and call me. I don't care what it is, you call me and talk to me." And I could do the same, any problem we had.... She was helping us learn to work together as a family ... about the eighth grade, he made a big turnaround like night to day. Just like once it was night and all of a sudden it was day.*
>
> ∼ Parent of a child with emotional and behavioral disorder

Several chapters in this book describe the development of service delivery systems for children with emotional and behavioral disorders (EBD). Most of these programs have been presented from the perspectives of administrators and staff. How do the parents of children with EBD experience these programs? While most recent developments in service delivery claim to be responsive to parents and siblings, we were interested in hearing directly from parents whether or not services have become family friendly. In a family-friendly service system, parents perceive that staff care about their children and families and are accessible to both children and parents in times of need. Responsive professionals also help families learn how to handle their own problems in crisis, and they have the expertise to provide appropriate treatment. This chapter presents the results of extensive interviews with parents of children with EBD. The interviews were conducted in order to elicit parents' perceptions of the professionals and services they have encountered, as well as to examine the impact of changes in the child services system on families.

Chapters 9 and 10 describe the development and implementation in Virginia of the Comprehensive Services Act for At Risk Children and Families (CSA). This legislative action sought to change a system of services that was provided through compartmentalized agencies and supported the placement of large numbers of children in residential care to a family-friendly system of care designed to provide cost-effective, integrated, holistic services within the home and community.

This chapter presents parents' perspectives on the changes—viewing through parents' eyes the old service system and the evolving CSA system. The information presented was obtained from across the state of Virginia from 122 parents of children with EBD. These parents participated in three qualitative studies that used extensive, in-depth, individual interviews and focus groups to elicit information about utilization, barriers and supports to access, and satisfaction with services. After spending more than 500 hours with these parents and an equal amount of time analyzing the data they shared, I am convinced that the best way of presenting this information is to let parents tell about their own experiences. To this end, I have used representative excerpts from interviews with the parents. The names of parents and children have been changed to protect their privacy.

The studies show that under the CSA plan, heartening progress has been achieved in making services meet the needs of families and children more adequately. They also show that while families do not wish to return to pre-CSA days, many report positive pre-CSA experiences with individual treatment providers, as demonstrated in the quote cited above from a mother discussing a pre-CSA experience. The anecdotal evidence from the parents interviewed indicates that positive change is taking place and that Virginia is moving away from the agency-oriented, residential-care-oriented ways of old, though the road is bumpy and the journey continues.

∿

DIFFERENT DRUMMERS: COPING WITH SEPARATE AND DIFFERENT SERVICES

The pre-CSA lack of service coordination among education, mental health, and juvenile justice (a CSA target) often left parents unsure of what problems their children had and who to turn to for help. Different agencies held different views of a child's problems and gave recommendations or took action based on these views. Consider Ms. Jackson, the single mother of a fourteen-year-old daughter, Gwendolyn, who is diagnosed as bipolar, and a son who is sixteen. The family lives in an inner-city neighborhood. In the following paragraphs, Ms. Jackson talks about her experiences when Gwendolyn first began having problems. As is often the case, Gwendolyn's disability was seen first as a school problem. It was only through Ms. Jackson's persistence in looking for help that the real problem was revealed.

> *She kept walking out of school and walking the halls and always smart to the teachers and stuff, so the principal got tired of her and kicked her out. She used to go out of the house at two o'clock, three o'clock in the morning, so I got scared for her and that's why I got a court of law in it.*
>
> *I had been asking for help. I asked for help from the school and they didn't tell me anything. When I first went to juvenile for help with [my son], this one lady there be telling me that they couldn't help him. I had to wait until he get in trouble before he could get help. I was mad. I was getting ready to. . . . But I didn't want to go to jail. The only thing they asked him was do we have underwears, do we have a T-shirt, do we have a toothbrush. She say, "Don't worry about it. We have it next door," then send him on home.*
>
> *Later, he had one probation officer who really helped him so I went to her and she told me to take Gwendolyn to mental health. The lady there, she asked a lot of questions and stuff. Want to know about your love life and all of that mess. They be nosey, nosey people. They want to know what I am doing, how me and my friend get along. It just irritated me so we didn't go back.*
>
> *Gwen didn't get help until [she went into a psychiatric hospital] and they found out she was bipolar and put her on Lithium. Big change. Big change.*

The separation of services, the personal and professional orientation of agencies and staff, and funding complications often meant that whether a child got appropriate services depended primarily on the determination of the parents, the expertise of available professional staff, and the community where they lived. Families could easily find themselves in need of a service offered by one agency, only to find they were ineligible because their child did not fit the category under which the service was offered. Conversely, they could also receive services from multiple agencies that offered multiple and often conflicting prescriptions for the best way to handle problems.

The rules separating services within a single agency frustrated Ms. Dixon, a middle-aged, single, African-American woman who works in financial accounting and is caretaker and legal guardian of her thirteen-year-old nephew who is diagnosed as having Dandy Walker syndrome with related emotional and behavioral problems and mental retardation. Assisting her with caretaking duties is her spry, seventy-plus-year-old mother who also lives in the home.

From the very first of having James, I constantly looked for things out in the community, like with social services or whatever, that I thought would help James and also help myself. What I was looking for too was a support group, a parent support group that I thought would be very helpful to me. To me it was the support—I thought I needed that. And to this day I'm still looking for that support.

Right after I got James, I saw this article in the paper about a training that was going on for parents that were taking care of children like James. So I called the lady and asked her, 'cause what I wanted to do was get involved in that training class. James came from the treatment center and it was going to be difficult to handle him, so I felt like I needed training in order to handle him. So I called. Everything that the article said fit me except for one thing: I did not have one of the children that they wanted to find a place for. I was sorta like a foster home would be, or adoptive parents, about knowing how to handle him. I mean everything fit except for that one thing and I was turned down from the training because of that. They had certain children that was evidently in the care of the state and they wanted to see them placed and they were willing to train these people in how to work with these children. So then they could put them in that home. My child was not one of the ones they were looking to place. They only wanted to train certain people. I really put a lot of pressure on that lady that day because I didn't accept the fact that I didn't qualify, I wanted to know why I didn't qualify. I felt quite disappointed. I felt that I needed this as much as other people do.

The training Ms. Dixon refers to was being offered by her community's department of social service. As a parent whose child was at home, she did not fit the categorical requirements of being a foster or adoptive parent. I first met Ms. Dixon and her mother when James was hospitalized following a crisis and they were having difficulty finding the services they needed in order to bring him home. Throughout my contact with them during their lengthy efforts to locate appropriate services for James, I never heard these determined women speak of an out-of-home placement, and it was clear that they were focused on finding a way to keep him at home.

Although foster and adoptive parents of children with emotional and behavioral disabilities were recognized as requiring such assistance as training, respite care, and additional pay, these same services were not available to parents to help them keep their children at home. Ironically, the department of social services had been involved with James's family during the time that his custody was transferred from his mother to Ms. Dixon, but since Ms. Dixon was a relative and James was not in the custody of the agency, the only services provided were those related to the custody issue. These services were separate from foster-care and adoption services, and clients who qualified for services in one area were not routinely eligible for services from another, even within the same agency.

This categorical structure was also true in mental health, as Ms. Dixon was shortly to find out—in an episode that easily could have ended tragically.

When he left the treatment center it was up to me to find a doctor, go to a doctor, and naturally we stuck with a neurological doctor. James was here at home, he was on a medication, and it did not work the same way it did at the treatment center. Instead of keeping him from being aggressive, it seemed to make him more aggressive.

This medicine wasn't working. I tried to contact the treatment center and ask the doctor there what I should do. He said he couldn't help, that I had to go to a doctor in the community. In the meantime, we are waiting to go see the neurological doctor, and he is so booked up that it might be a month or so before you get to see him. It really left it up to me to try to handle this problem at home, the side effects that J was having. So basically I tried to make decisions the best I could, but really I was working with something that I really didn't know.

Eventually it wound up that things were not working so well, and I kept talking to the neurologist and he said just take him off the medicine. What I found was interesting, too. I had raised this issue with the neurologist of this medicine having side effects. He was like, "No, this medicine doesn't have side effects." After a while, you realize, when we have problems we go back to the neurologist and he would tell us that basically he was out of his field. He only deals from a neurological and physical standpoint, not from a mental and emotional standpoint, and that's basically what that medicine was for.

Okay. So what happened? Things got so much out of hand here. James was on the medication. He must have been having side effects. He would become aggressive. He said numerous times that he wanted to hurt somebody, so he was like a time bomb. One night he had a string and kept saying, "I'm going to hurt somebody, hurt somebody." So I'm thinking what am I going to do. That morning he took it a step further. He actually got a knife, and my mother and I had to quickly restrain him, and it took us both to handle him, and we couldn't even make a call for help because we had to hold him. It took us a while to even figure out what we were going to do. So there again, I wasn't really qualified to handle it.

Hospital and residential facility staff provided treatment only to children in their programs. Discharge from the program required a change in doctors. Further complicating matters for Ms. Dixon was the fact that mental health and mental retardation services in the community functioned as separate departments within the same agency. A child was treated under the service related to his or her primary diagnosis. For James, this meant mental retardation services. Unfortunately, not only did mental retardation services not include psychiatric care, but children with mental retardation as their primary diagnosis were not eligible for mental health services.

> *We had been told before that psychiatrists don't treat mentally retarded children. We had been sent to two different psychiatrists and that was what we were told—that they were sorry that they couldn't do anything for him because a child like this cannot relate to us how he is feeling emotionally so that we can treat him.*
>
> *So our next obstacle was trying to find one that would be willing to take James on as a client. We went directly from the [psychiatric hospital] to [community] mental health. That's how I found out that mental retardation don't have a doctor [a child psychiatrist] but mental health do. So I pushed the issue of the fact that he had a need for a doctor and that they should go ahead and serve him even though he was mentally retarded. So we had to deal with that. . . .*
>
> *When I told them at the emergency room [after the knife incident] what I had been through I just said, "I don't want to go through this no more. I don't want to put this child through what we have put him through no more. We are going to have to do something and no more will I take this." They admitted that we had been handled wrong. They apologized to me. She said, "I am sorry about what happened to you." I says, "What happened was they let him out of the [psychiatric hospital] and nobody followed up with how we were doing at home." I was left on my own.*

Parents confronting the difficulties created by the separate service systems were embarking on what Joseph Campbell might refer to as a heroine's journey (Campbell, 1990) to find a treasure: appropriate treatment and services. The women's responses to these difficulties were typical of heroines. They confronted agencies responsible for services; when they did not find satisfactory answers in one place they continued their search in another; and they tried to handle the problems themselves. Only the strong survive the heroine's journey.

MEA CULPA: THE BLAME GAME

In addition to frustrations arising from the separation of services, parents suffered personal pain from the effects of a long-standing belief among both professionals and the general public that parents were to blame for children's emotional and behavioral problems. These beliefs created an additional burden of guilt and often meant enduring accusations that were hard to refute and treatment interventions aimed at correcting parents. The following account by Ms. Allen, a Caucasian mother from a rural area of Virginia whose ten-year-old son is diagnosed with Attention Deficit Hyperactivity Disorder (ADHD), shows how both parents and children are blamed for emotional disabilities.

> *The school isn't going to tell you what your options are. The school is not going to come and tell you your child is attention deficit disordered. They're going to tell you "It's your fault." "You don't teach respect." "You don't stress education." [My child] didn't get any testing until he was in fifth grade. It turned into a big mushroomed argument. Like I told them, "You have seen the same behaviors year after year. Why do you think we're having the same behaviors? He knows his spelling words perfectly at home then gets here, draws a total blank, and gets an F. That's my fault? Maybe it's your fault. What's up here that's holding him back?"*
>
> *The papers they would send home were word for word, symptoms of attention deficit disorder, but they knew nothing about attention deficit disorder. It's much easier to put a label on them [the kids]. "They're a trouble maker." "They don't want to do." "They're lazy." The principal just picks up the phone [and calls the parent]. "You have to come and get your son." I would like to find a place that would deal with him and not pick up the phone and say, "Come and get him." That's easy to do. That takes the problem away from [the school], but he is not learning.*

Because school is such an important part of a child's life on a day-to-day basis, problems in school are the most troubling to parents and tend to be prominent in their stories even though the blame game is by no means confined to the educational arena. Mental health literature is replete with references to disorders and disabilities whose causes are at least in part ascribed to mothers, fathers, and "dysfunctional families." Further, parents confront this attitude daily in the community where day-care centers, recreational programs, and neighborhood play groups exclude their children.

SOPHIE'S CHOICE

The parents who were part of the three studies had maintained their children in the home in spite of the difficulties they encountered with treatment and services. However, during the twenty years prior to the CSA, children were placed steadily and increasingly out of the home in residential and hospital programs. Almost all of these children were in the custody of either the department of social services or the department of corrections. Although no statistics show the number of children with emotional disabilities whose custody was transferred from their parent(s) to these departments primarily for the purpose of placement in residential care, some studies do show this was a prevalent practice. Ms. Jordan, a parent in one of the focus groups, described her feelings about this situation.

> *In order to get services before [CSA], your children had to either be on special education or foster care and I'm here to tell you there have been times when I wanted to make them foster-care kids. You get upset, you get frustrated, you get angry. The system tells you if they are foster-care kids they can get anything they need and so you're tempted.*

Because community-based services were so often lacking, caring professionals had little alternative except to recommend expensive residential treatment. But residential treatment was beyond the private means of most people, so parents were presented with an American version of "Sophie's Choice." Either give up children to the custody of the state, thus opening the door to residential treatment at state expense, or retain custody and keep children in the home environment, thereby effectively denying them the help that only residential placement could provide. Ms. Bond was encouraged to put her six grandchildren in foster care but had refused this option.

> *I had my grandchildren, all six of them. It was so hard for me to care for these kids and they were telling me, "You'll come out better making yourself a foster mother." The catch here is you can give your kids up and the fact that, you know, I was afraid to do it. I wouldn't do it. . . . They told me that if I were to make myself a foster parent then I would have funds to get services and treatment for these kids. But there were no guarantees that I would get to keep all these kids. . . . Seems like they like to break up families and all that kind of stuff.*

Other parents made the painful decision to go to court and ask that the state take custody of their children. Only later would they realize the full impact of this decision. Somebody else would be making decisions about where their children were placed, what kind of treatment they received, when they could visit their children, or when the children could visit at home. Ms. Harrison was one of these parents.

> *Shortly after she went into the hospital the first time, I lost my insurance and I certainly couldn't pay for it and the only way to get funding was if we turned over her custody. . . . That was very scary. I felt like I was losing complete control of what happened to her and she still wasn't improving. I also*

felt pushed into a corner. Sometimes things would happen and she would get injured and stuff and I know that she could make people very angry and I think some of the injuries were probably staff people fighting with her.

Many residential programs operated under the belief that the parents were to blame for their children's problems and so they discouraged parental involvement in the children's treatments. Many also believed that in order for children to adjust to residential care, it was necessary to cut ties with the parents while children adjusted to a new environment. This meant no contact with parents and family for predetermined periods of time that ranged from a few weeks to a couple of months. Even after contact was allowed, the frequency of visits was controlled by staff.

The results of these practices are painfully obvious. Parents and children frequently lost contact with each other. Children's behavior often got worse, and they were moved from place to place as staff in residential programs decided that the children had received "maximum benefits" from a particular program or that the children were unable to benefit from the program. Those children who were returned home found it difficult to adjust to home and community living because they had become institutionalized.

POINTS OF LIGHT

We have heard the parents' perspective on the problems that the CSA was designed to address, but the picture of services pre-CSA is not totally bleak. Although difficult and painful experiences are often the most memorable, parents reported positive experiences as well. These reports included a variety of services, but they invariably focused on attributes that have come to be known as "family friendly."

David was a youth with a long history of emotional and behavioral disorders that included such diagnoses as learning disabled, intermittent explosive disorder, and ADHD. In the quote that opened this chapter, his mother, Ms. Roberts, had high praise for the counselor who came to their home. She also felt that a family group run by the local mental health agency had been beneficial to both her and David.

That was a great help. We used to go every Wednesday, David and I would go. I think it started at six and lasted until nine. That was another big help. That came out of mental health too. . . . They talked to you and told you about nurturing and how to talk to one another. And if you are angry how to keep from acting out. So many helpful things they told us in there, so many ideas and things that we can bring home like giving quality time, families getting together and sharing and doing things. He [the facilitator] really gave us a big help. It was a class that was done in two parts. The first part they would take the parents all together and another lady would take the teenagers. The other half they would bring everybody together and we shared our views. Maybe it was in a painting, maybe we talked, maybe we told different family problems of our childhood, and all that together it was good.

David and I did it for a year. I'm saying a year. We did it like from September to June. Then the man left. They had a great man there and David loved talking to him.

Relationships with professionals and the ability to contact a treatment provider when needed were frequently mentioned when a parent discussed services, as was the absence of a trusted professional to talk to when a problem left a parent feeling alone and unable to prevent a crisis, as with Ms. Dixon and James. Conversely, having a professional provide the option to call for help when needed, or even to encourage a call, promoted an attitude that the professional was an ally, as with David's mother. This notion is somewhat at odds with the traditional professional view that such openness either promotes "client dependence" or crosses the boundaries of a professional relationship.

In the following excerpt, a mother talks about being "bonded" to a professional. From this parent's perspective, this was a bond between two people who had worked together and successfully handled a situation, as it might be between any two coworkers.

She has been the best social worker. She wasn't even in the field to handle kids but they gave her this case. She put herself on the case. She used to be one of the top persons and she took the job over. She was, she is, so good, I had just got so bonded to her, and in fact she had became too close on the case, so involved in the case, that they wanted her off. But she has been there for Brian, I guess because she has a child too with special needs. So, she was just so understanding and very pushy to get what I needed and very understanding.

The existence of "points of light" helped to shape the objectives of the CSA and point the way toward family-friendly services and away from the historically child-focused system.

WHEN CHANGE WAS GOOD, IT WAS VERY, VERY GOOD

By focusing on management and organizational problems, the objectives of the Comprehensive Services Act provided a structure to foster a change in the attitudes and beliefs of both parents and professionals, to promote a customer-friendly climate in agencies, and to give parents a real choice about treatment and services for their children and families. Among numerous changes that ensued passage of the CSA, one of the most visible and dramatic was the way in which parents accessed services. Each community established a multidisciplinary team comprised of agency and parent representatives (Family Assessment and Planning Teams [FAPT]) to determine service needs of families and children and either to locate or design appropriate services to meet those needs.

Some parents reported that the ideals of the CSA were fully realized in their communities. Others reacted with equal enthusiasm and also made suggestions for further improvements. Ms. Bradford, mother of a teenage son who had been diagnosed with emotional disabilities when he was six years old, described her very positive experience by comparing her experiences before and after the CSA changes.

Before the FAPT team [we used to go to] special ed meetings. We felt outnumbered at these meetings because the administration was all represented and we were the ones coming into that. It was sorta like you all sing the same song, we had that feeling—sorta outnumbered, it was a formality of being there. They controlled the money. They made all the decisions. They didn't want to spend the money. They would just say we want to try this or that, and we spent over a year trying so many things that were constantly failing. We had all these failures and the child regressed to the point that he had to be put in residential. I never felt that was necessary had we gotten the proper answers or the proper attention at the time.

He came back [home from residential] after two-and-a-half years. We go to the FAPT team and it's a different answer. You really felt welcome, not an imposition or being there taking up their valuable time. You had many avenues on the FAPT team that I didn't even know existed. I would feel like I could go to them and lay out a problem and say this is what I see, this is what I think might help, and I had people that were really trying to resolve the problem. They were all there collectively, as a group. They could talk to each other and say "What do you think about this" [and another one] would say "We have anger control groups in our agency and I can see about getting him in that program." Well I wouldn't know anything about anger control. So there were more avenues open because there was a broader dialogue within the community that could bring up what they could support, what they knew about. They were there to resolve a problem, to address the problem within the community resources.

The school situation in the past, to me it was a very hostile environment and [the FAPT] was a very supportive, more nurturing environment to the parents.

In order to implement the CSA, it was necessary to create services within the community that would support families in maintaining their children at home. Both private and state agencies began offering parent training, respite care, in-home services, and day treatment. In addition, both types of agencies also created, in some communities, such out-of-home placements as therapeutic foster care and small group homes. The gatekeepers to the services were the FAPT, who made recommendations for services to another multidisciplinary committee, the Community Planning and Management Team (CPMT), responsible for funding. Parents seeking services were referred to the FAPT by one of the participating agencies and attended the FAPT meetings but not the CPMT meetings. Theoretically, this change promoted a partnership between professionals and parents and gave the parents active voice in planning services for their children and families.

What Ms. Bradford described in the above quote was the CSA principles in action: the parent-professional partnership, integrated services, and children at home with their parents. Ms. Long, a young mother only recently introduced to services for children with EBD, was also happy with the services and the FAPT, with only one caveat, that her child's problems had to reach a crisis point before she knew about available services.

> *I didn't know they had all this out here until he had to be sent to Richmond [to a psychiatric hospital located 200 miles from home] and then they got a meeting together quick before he came back home from Richmond.*
>
> *I was just amazed at how much they could do for you actually. When I first went to [FAPT] they're sitting around a desk and I was nervous and everything and I didn't know exactly what was going to happen. As we got into it I found out what they can do for you. Now they are giving my son, which is seven years old, giving him respite. A counselor keeps him every other week. That helps out a lot. I was all alone by myself. . . . I found out that they can do a lot for you. . . .*
>
> *I didn't know they could do all these things for you because I had to get to a point where I was desperate. When I got there they helped me out and it was amazing what all they could do for you.*

Mrs. Schmidt, a strong advocate for her son and a leader in parent support groups in her area, was enthusiastic about the services but found the process long and arduous.

> *When you're dealing with a child and if it's crisis oriented or you've just been dealing with it so long and you need to see some kind of service in place, it just sometimes seems like it can take months. I know with my son's education placement, we started that process in April or May and didn't get the final approval (from FAPT) until the Friday before Labor Day, that afternoon in*

an emergency session, that they would approve. That was a four-month process of yes, no, maybe. That's too long for me as a parent, and I'm the adult, that was away too long for my ten-year-old child. That process I would like to see expedited in some way so it's a little bit smoother and you don't have to bounce and wave and feel like you're going into court and need a lawyer.

AND WHEN IT WAS BAD...

The response of professionals and communities to the CSA varied from one locality to another as did the quality and quantity of services and the reactions of parents. The positive experiences reported by parents post-CSA show that change is possible and the process of change worth the effort. Other experiences seemed to prove the old maxim "The more things change the more they stay the same." As the CSA services became better established in communities, both professionals and parents sought to utilize the new opportunities for children, and the requests for services increased well beyond the funding. Once more, communities resorted to the restrictive eligibility criteria of first serving children who were in special education or foster care. These were the "mandated kids," so-called because federal funding streams were tied to services for this population. Unfortunately, after the needs of this group were served, little if any money was left to meet the needs of other children and their families and none was left for prevention. For many families, the service system issues post-CSA were the same as pre-CSA: personal and professional orientation of agencies and staff, access to services, and funding. However, families were becoming more defensive of both their children and themselves. They responded to denials of access to services and negative attitudes with anger and action.

Ms. Campbell, a divorced, Caucasian mother from the mountain area whose fifteen-year-old son is diagnosed with Oppositional Defiant Disorder, tried to give the FAPT a clear picture of the problem by using a technique that professional literature would refer to as "experiential learning."

[My son] is an oppositional defiant, and he refuses medication. I would love to give him medication. I have had people on the FAPT team say that maybe we can't be referred to the money team unless he is on medication. I say, "Well, this kid is bigger than I am. Do I hold him and force medicine down his throat?"

I tell the FAPT team all the time, "You have no idea what you are talking about unless you've been there with one of these kids." So I brought mine to the team one day, to the meeting with us. I mean it was a real eye-opener because his oppositional defiance was just in full bloom that day. They saw it and they were not impressed. I was surprised that they didn't refuse to see us all together anymore.

FROM BLAME TO SHAME

Parents who were enthusiastic about the CSA changes described an attitude of openness and caring on the part of professionals. Others parents were critical of what they perceived to be a continuing "family-unfriendly" atmosphere. To be sure, parents did not report any statements by agencies or staff post-CSA that openly blamed parents for causing their children's problems. Instead, their stories indicated that the old blame game seemed to have become the shame game: Parents should be able to take care of their own children. No longer willing to accept this criticism, parents openly began to confront it. Mothers in one of the focus groups spoke candidly about their feelings.

I think some of the people [need to be] a little bit more humane in their treatment of parents and to be a little bit more empathetic and understanding that we are talking about the lives of our most cherished possessions and we are not money-grubbing folks who want a free ride.

There are special guidelines, and they act like they have to take the money out of their pocket, is what I thought. . . . They were acting like the money was coming personally from one person or from a group of people. . . . The person looked like it was their money it was coming from. We are human beings, and if I feel humiliated, and if I feel intimidated and put down, I'm wondering how other parents who haven't a clue about this process may feel in these situations. I think they need to be more sensitive.

The story of Ms. Forrest, a professionally educated, African-American mother of a fourteen-year-old son diagnosed with Asberger's syndrome, details the range of emotions parents experience when they work within the system to get help for their children.

Ms. Forrest: *I was sharing how stressful it was trying to get William focused. It takes an hour to get him focused enough to get dressed so that he can get on a school bus at six-twenty with a pop tart and a carton of milk in his book bag. Then he has to sit on another bus, go to the high school, get off the bus that took him from home, and get on another bus that takes him to the middle school, and then go back across town to [his alternative school place-*

ment]. So someone said, "Can't you just drive him?" I was angry at that point because I had been to so many meetings and felt that the system was jerking us around and I said, "No. I cannot drive him. Physically I cannot drive him. Financially I cannot drive him." I felt that at times it was almost like if we beat up on her enough she will just take him out of the school system and put him in a private school. If she gets tired enough of this bus situation she will just transport him herself. It's almost like I am being discriminated against.

Facilitator: *Because you are black?*

Ms. Forrest: *No, because I am a professional person. It is a very lonely and very—I don't know what word I can find to describe what I feel in those meetings. Discompassion at one level.*

I've asked the question about why can't I go to the level where the decisions are made, the CPMT. Is there a policy that says I can't go? And nobody can give me an answer.

I did reach a point where I decided I had to pick my battles because the stress that I was feeling warned me that I could go over the edge and then I couldn't help William. By just constantly fighting about something or meeting, I couldn't work, I was constantly having to call patients and reschedule appointments or cancel because of having to go to these meetings and I had no choice, I had to go to those meetings. Even though they would say to me you really don't have to come.

But so many positive things had occurred [such as] them providing mentoring services.

ACCESS TO SERVICES: SOPHIE'S NEW CHOICES

While post-CSA children with the most serious behavioral problems were still finding their way into state custody via either the department of social service or the department of corrections, parents whose children had not reached this stage or who were determined to keep their kids at home reported continuing frustrations. Services existed that could help children and their families, but they were not accessible. Choices now ranged from giving up and accepting the status quo, to fighting for the help their children needed, to creating their own services for their children. A couple of parents described feelings of helplessness.

It's so much a stark difference between listening to her [a foster parent] say all of the services that are already in place for her child, as a foster-care child, and the rest of us who are begging for and basically going without.

Things may be better now but it's like going before a firing squad every time you go [to FAPT]. To me it makes me sick on my stomach, I guess because you're in that position. You go to the FAPT team and—I mean I qualify for absolutely nothing.

Other parents chose to fight the system and were skillful in presenting their cases to the FAPT. Ms. Taylor is an African-American mother who has worked in human services and is knowledgeable about the system. Her child met the mandated eligibility criteria but needed services that still were not available. The use of persuasive arguments did not alter the outcome.

I am still trying to get services for my children. I have three children that have been diagnosed with SED [Serious Emotional Disabilities]. One has a very serious mental health problem that wound him up in the juvenile justice system, I have one that I'm trying to keep from getting into the juvenile justice system, and a daughter who is mainly behavioral problems.

All three of these children have witnessed and experienced violence. They saw, each of them has seen, at least three people shot and killed and one stabbing death, which I think in part contributed to their SED problem. When my oldest boy first began to exhibit his problems, I cannot even begin to tell you the number of agencies, organizations, people that I called for help. We'd gone to the FAPT teams and we'd not gotten services.

I was told the last time I went before the FAPT team that yes, my child was a mandated child but the services were not. And I don't quite know how to make that connect. It's extremely frustrating when you have a child that you know needs help with services and you can't get them. And you come up with all these reasons why your child can't get the services.

What we were asking for, for this child, he's in a special ed program, he's a SED child, and we wanted him to have after-school counseling services. We wanted alcohol and drug abuse counseling services, and we wanted some type of recreational services. In other words, we wanted to keep him busy. But those services were not forthcoming.

Now I was told if I put him in [an alternative school] that some of those services would be available there. But not every environment is appropriate for every child and at the time we, and when I say we I'm talking about his therapist, his psychologist, and his psychiatrist, we all in unison did not feel [the alternative school] was the most appropriate placement for this child at that time. Since we were not willing to accept their recommendations we got no services.

Other parents gave up on the FAPTs and the CSA but did not give up on their children. They were creative in finding the best ways they could to provide their children with the experiences and services they needed. The action Ms.

Roberts took was not typical of what other parents were able to do, but her determination and spirit are representative of all the parents we interviewed. Ms. Roberts, who is responsible for our opening quote, is a middle-aged widow with a life-threatening heart disease. She and David, her sixteen-year-old son, live in a rural area. David is learning disabled and has had various mental health diagnoses, including ADHD and Intermittent Explosive Disorder. Ms. Roberts has used her problem-solving skills and a lot of ingenuity to provide her son with the help she believes he needs. While this often means finding the right professional help, if none is available she finds other means. One example of this was her provision of "vocational education." When school staff told her they did not have a vocational educational program, Ms. Roberts created an "individualized" program for David.

> Ms. Roberts: *Well one thing I believe in is working. That was something that we have always done. We were taught to work. I didn't like to when I was a child but I found out since I got older that is one of the best things that you can do. It's a healthy thing for you. So as soon as he got old enough to push a grass cutter, I started him working. Then I would pay him something.*
>
> *Then he started getting SSI [Social Security benefits]. He doesn't know he gets that. Now I used to give him ten dollars every month and just tell him, "That is yours to spend when you want to." I don't know how we are going to work it this summer 'cause I am going to try to work him again this summer from here. I'm going to have to find somebody to work with him this summer. I have worked with him each summer, and since he was old enough to work I have taken him to work each time. I did that clean up until last year. I have some friends that know him and know me, and I went to those friends and asked them, 'cause sometimes things are hard for him to judge. Like cutting grass, he might go and leave a streak in it or something like that. I asked them if they would allow him to cut the grass for them and I would pay most of it. Most of them agreed to it 'cause they were getting it for little or nothing, so they let him come and work. So each afternoon, every day, we would take a yard and he would go and do that. I had to go with him, and then I would pay him and he would be able to save his money.*
>
> *Last year now I talked to a man that had a field, a soybean field, which the weeds wouldn't have been pulled 'cause he wasn't going to pull them. I asked him if he'd let us pull the weeds and I paid David to pull the weeds. He'd go out there in the afternoon and work four or five hours. We'd wait till it cooled off or else early in the morning and we would do that work and then come on home. That way he'd done half a day's work.*

Facilitator: *What were you looking to teach him?*

Ms. Roberts: *Responsibility. Responsibility. And that nothing doesn't come in this world from nothing. You don't get a thing in this world for free, and he should learn to work for it. That is the most important thing in the world. And it is healthy for him. Keeps his mind and keeps him out of trouble. I'm hoping for all that.*

So this year I have got to talk to another man I know and see if he will take him on 'cause I won't be able to go with him this year 'cause I'm not even driving right now [because of her heart condition]. I don't know but I'm going to see if somebody will take him on this year, and maybe if he doesn't work but a half a day, certain hours and certain times that he works because some of the things he forgets. Like putting his food in the oven, then he might forget about it. Which all of us do at times, some a little more so than others.

So if he works with you, someone has to sorta pay attention to certain things that he might forget. Like painting. The house was in real bad shape and my daughter got some paint and they came home one day and they went out, my son-in-law and all the children, they went out and they painted the house for me to make it look a little better. My son-in-law left David painting and he done the greatest job painting. So now I know that he can paint. So I am going to ask for a paint job if somebody will hire him doing that.

Ms. Roberts represents every parent who uses all the energy and effort possible to give her child what he will need to function as an adult. Further, she represents the American-idealized characteristics of independence and self-reliance. Interwoven in her story is also another American version of "Sophie's Choice." If her child is denied the education to which he is entitled, the parent does the best she can on her own.

When we talked to David, he listed two of his main worries: (1) What happens when he has to apply for a job and "they" find out he can't read, and (2) If something happens to his mother, what will happen to him?

David has many creative talents. He also plays inspired chess, displays excellent verbal and thinking skills, and gets along well with other people. Will he have the opportunity to choose a future career based on his interests?

IN RETROSPECT

We recently recontacted some of the parents who appear in this chapter to see what had happened to them and their children since the studies.

Ms. Schwartz accessed the educational program her son needed.

Whatever they paid, and I know it was a big chunk of money, for my child to go to day treatment, it was well worth it, well worth it. Because he is able to manage himself better, he is able to control himself better. My child is not cured by any means. My son's case manager said, "He's not cured. We've never cured a child with Attention Deficit Disorder." But he's developed more coping skills and management skills for dealing with [ADHD]. My child will be in special education until he graduates. I'm fine with that and he's fine with that . . . if he doesn't have to go away—as long as he can stay in public schools.

Ms. Dixon and her now seventy-seven-year-old mother continue to care for James and so far have been successful in their efforts to get services for him— but not without some difficulties.

We went to [FAPT] and the caseworker helped us to get a couple of things that we wanted. My mother brought up the suggestion of a male role model because he is a male among females. Basically that day we had a pretty lengthy discussion and I simply again laid my cards on the table . . . so we got assigned a counselor . . . and this person really addressed many issues with James— being aggressive, him needing to obey the parents, the rules or whatever, how they behaved in school. They covered a lot of things. This gentleman has really been excellent with James. He's brought James out.

Right now what has happened is the last time I went to an FAPT team, what they had been doing was approving the service for three months. This time, due to the money situation they are facing right now, I was informed by the caseworker that the FAPT right now has a limit on services and we had already went over our limit. It's a $6,000 limit. But there is certain circum- stances which they will approve of more.

So we had to go to FAPT and . . . they gave us a month to look at alternative things we could do for James and take him out of this in-home service. James has been doing so well with this in-home service . . . I tried to tell the FAPT how James is a disability child and his problems are not temporary, they are permanent.

Basically this type of service where a male comes in and is involved with a male child is very important, very beneficial. Sometimes it makes a difference to whether they make it or not.

Ms. Roberts has been less successful with the system. She believes that David will leave school when he turns eighteen. He did not learn how to read, and he sees no reason to continue in school. The family continues as it always has, providing him support as a valued family member. Just as they took steps to provide special education services, to the best of their ability, they are now looking for job opportunities for him.

Family-friendly services is an idea whose time has come. Validated and defined by the CSA, this idea was sent to communities and professionals to be given form. The form that evolved varied from one location to another as did parents' reactions to the changes. Through the activities sanctioned by the CSA, parents became more knowledgeable about EBD and the service system and better able to act as partners with professionals in the treatment of their children with EBD. When such a partnership was invited, the stories reported by parents reflected a renewed energy and enthusiasm from both sides of the partnership and also revealed the parents' satisfaction with the services and the outcomes.

Parents, however, also became less willing to accept either blame or shame or settle for a "Sophie's Choice." As with Ms. Taylor, who was denied recreational programs and substance-abuse treatment for her son under the CSA process, these parents want the same opportunities for their children with emotional disorders as the community provides for other children.

Regardless of the attitudes they encounter or the services they receive, parents have responded to the changes and the partial successes of the CSA by continuing the business of being a parent, seeing to it that their children have what they need to grow into functioning adults. Some parents have continued to push the system for needed services, with more or less success; some have transferred custody of their children to the state; and others have given up on the CSA and the community and found other ways to help their children.

POINTS TO PONDER

1. The involvement of parents in the planning and provision of services for their children and families has become a critical standard in assessing quality of treatment and services. However, the interpretation of the term "involvement" varies widely among both professionals and parents. How would you define parent involvement? How would you set up a process that promotes parent involvement? What obstacles might you encounter?

2. If there is to be a partnership between parents and professionals in the treatment of children with emotional and behavioral disabilities, what are the roles of each? How do the traditional roles of clients and professionals support and interfere with a partnership?

3. Based on your reading and experiences both in and out of the children's services field, what individual and system changes are necessary for a real partnership between parents and professionals?

4. Some of the parents quoted in this chapter discussed being confronted with a version of "Sophie's Choice"—having to give up custody of a child in order to obtain services or keeping a child and being denied access to needed services. Discuss the impact of this dilemma on parents and consider strategies for providing a full complement of services to children while still maintaining custody with the parents. Take into account that this situation has been created, in part, by the lack of sufficient resources to provide services for all children in need.

CLASSROOM TO COMMUNITY

Applying the Concepts of Change

- Select an agency that provides services to children with emotional and behavioral disabilities and describe the role of the parents in treatment and services. Assess the strengths and weaknesses of this agency in relation to the way in which it involves parents. Describe how parental involvement could be increased and describe the impact of this greater involvement on effectiveness and outcomes.

CHAPTER 13

Young Worker's Perspective

LEARNING THE ROPES

YOUNG PEOPLE ENTERING HUMAN SERVICES

> *Members of Generation X have much to offer your organization. They have the team-building, information-processing skills needed in today's workplace, and they're eager to make a difference in the world. They are energetic, philanthropic, and enterprising. As they make their mark on the American landscape, your ability to meet their needs will determine your success in the marketplace. Your challenge is to tap into their creativity, spirit, vitality, diversity, and idealism to improve your organization.*
>
> ~ Mark A. Mitchell, Assistant Professor of Marketing
> ~ Robert Orwig, Assistant Professor of Management

C omplex issues are always involved when young people go to work in their first jobs after college. I am interested in exploring some of the issues particular to working in human services during this time of change and redesign. The bulk of this book focuses on the experiences of one person in the higher ranks of administration and management. In this chapter, I address the experience of younger workers in human services. These individuals approached their work from diverse backgrounds and held very different positions. None of the people interviewed took positions that were advertised as clerical in nature, but the spectrum of actual responsibilities was wide and always included that level of responsibility.

During recent years a great deal of definition and speculation have been generated about "Generation X." Some people define this generation as broadly as those born between 1961 and 1981, but the term is often used to define the group of people born between 1965 and 1978. Countless marketing schemes, films, studies, and the like have been created to define this generation of which I am a member. An inordinate amount of attention has been paid to the productivity (or supposed lack thereof) of a whole decade's worth of births that some have tried very hard to homogenize. After writing my own narrative about working as a young person in human services, I decided to investigate the experience of others in my generation, especially those who are direct service providers. By no means do I consider these interviews wholly representative of the experiences of young people working in human services. I selected a small cross section of individuals under thirty from different backgrounds who worked in various human services settings. I asked each person a series of questions concerning their training for this work, their treatment as young workers, and how this work affects their world view. Much of what I learned links directly to the factors mentioned in Chapters 1 and 2; all their experiences have been shaped by those factors: economics, technology, and politics. Each of these individuals entered the workforce in the current climate of human services. These interviewees served as direct service providers in organizations ranging from welfare-to-work reading programs to support networks for family members of children with rare diseases.

~

TRAINING: ON THE JOB AND OFF

All of the people I interviewed had pursued liberal arts degrees at the under-graduate level. I chose not to talk to people who had been educated or trained specifically for work in human services. I was interested particularly in find-ing out whether the various undergraduate experiences had provided any strong preparation—formal or informal—for working in human services. Several people had some informal training or had an inspiring experience at that level. Most individuals discovered that the skills necessary to do their work and the issues that arose could not have been anticipated by an under-graduate program.

Pat, who had first attended a large university where he did not do well aca-demically, finished his B.A. at a small college in a liberal arts setting. He was an English major and took no education classes, but he did complete a teach-ing internship at the college level at his own school.

I taught freshman core and remedial English. In addition to meeting every week with my adviser, I had two meetings a week with the core faculty and the tutoring faculty [adjunct and tenured faculty]. Most of my students were EOF [Education Opportunity Fund] students, so I had exposure to an underprivi-leged population early on. When I started teaching [reading in the welfare-to-work program], I was overwhelmed. I was dealing with a community that was entirely different from me. I was getting a lot of pressure to teach in a way that wasn't mine. The YWCA hired a consultant reading specialist who interviewed teaching candidates. She hired me and ended up giving me four fat books on reading theory and saying this is how you teach reading.

Pat added later that his the starting date of his course was delayed by three weeks because another group was occupying the designated space. His anecdote and many others I heard demonstrated the challenges facing human services workers. Limited resources required that Pat begin teaching without full training. He described the experience of teaching as valuable and believed that he helped his students learn to read, but he continued to be frustrated by the external factors that impeded their progress.

One woman I interviewed believed her church fellowship and volunteer work have been good training or education in human services because she learned to work with people in various capacities. As a sociology student at a university in the Northeast, Judith did an independent study in which she and another student designed a public service curriculum for residents in a college dorm. The program contained three major elements: education, community, and service. The next year the university implemented her design. She participated in a number of volunteer activities and took a course that required students to volunteer with organizations. Finally, the university she attended ran an experimental college in which students volunteered to teach. While Judith had no formal training in organizational behavior or human services, she graduated from this liberal arts institution with a solid foundation for work in the field.

Others approached the question from a more conceptual angle. I interviewed several individuals who cited their coursework in women's studies as the best academic preparation for this work. They spoke in broad terms about the basic ways in which students explore human behavior.

The curriculum that prepared me for human services work was found in my women's studies and sociology courses where I learned all of the basics about inequality, social structures, appreciation of difference, my own "unearned privileges," my role as insider or outsider, and so on. . . . Curriculum should contain all of those basics plus the ideas about why we don't always know what's best for the people we're "helping" and what role we need to take when working with different communities.

One advantage that many individuals in my age group have in entering human services is this "training" at the undergraduate level in diversity as it relates to race, class, gender, and sexuality. Jessica, who worked as a case manager for a national organization and as a program assistant in a small housing organization, felt that she had received this general theoretical preparation but had very little experience in applying the concepts. As part of her women's studies curriculum, she took several social science classes (anthropology, psychology, and sociology). I was interested in her reaction to this particular question because we had attended the same college and taken many of the same courses. She had coordinated workshops surrounding domestic and relationship violence during college, which taught her about maintaining nonjudgmental attitudes. However, the school's curriculum included no systematic introduction to the work in these fields.

I think my women's studies degree counted for getting my job. It gave me a greater general awareness [of the] complexities of issues surrounding women . . . confidence in my ability to work my way around and advocate for other people. Writing op-eds was helpful—short, terse, expressive, persuasive pieces. I took a community-organizing seminar but learned little—it was dry and inaccessible. We wrote papers about the theories, but I wanted more of an applied setting. I didn't understand the connections between the various issues.

Her desire for this training was echoed in interviews with others who believe that their only real training for work in human services was related to writing skills. It is difficult to know how to prepare students concentrating in such a wide array of subjects, especially at small colleges where students choose most of their courses without distribution requirements.

As a way of probing school preparation versus both formal and informal on-the-job training, I asked people to describe the skills they possessed before they entered this field and those they had to acquire. Once again, the responses were quite varied, ranging from the very technical to the more conceptual skills of listening, compassion, and problem solving.

[I] need to learn organization and documentation . . . sticking to one task . . . discipline . . . a couple of workshops and training sessions . . . advice from my coworkers, all of whom have been here a lot longer than I have [has helped]. The skills I had before were listening skills, a high level of compassion, nonjudgmental behavior, and basic grammar and usage. The ability to be persuasive, but I had to work on being confrontational sometimes. I did a lot of reading—I was there for over a month before I saw clients. Some things you can't understand until you are doing them. I have been asking coworkers, and I have meetings with my supervisor once a week.

Abby, who worked in an office of a national housing organization, emphasized the importance of understanding the influence of political factors on work in human services.

[I would have liked to have] a broad understanding of the relationships between nongovernmental nonprofits and city political structures and poli-

cies. I learned all this on the job. I came into the job with the ability to write
"grammatically correct" sentences—a skill I learned was respected by my
coworkers. I did not possess an understanding of the organization operating
within a larger social structure. I also knew nothing of fundraising, aside
from bake sales.

Judith, who worked as a residence manager for a group home for women
recovering from substance abuse, said that she relies daily on the knowledge
she gained during that year.

*I had a thorough understanding of larger socioeconomic factors that were
acting on the lives of the women that I was working with [from a seminar on
domestic violence]. What it didn't give me was viable cross-cultural relational
skills. [I] ended up realizing that I was not the right person for the job. My
training on the job was absolute immersion in twelve-step theory and practice. In retrospect, supervisors were overinvolved and codependent. [But I]
haven't come across any better organization for training.*

Pat added these thoughts:

*[I] needed to learn about public assistance programs. They [the students]
wanted to talk about issues. My boss was really supportive, but she was so
overwhelmed herself that we didn't have time to sit down and figure out
logistics. What [college] did do for me was prepare me to work with different
kinds of people. Let me look at the world and say I don't know what . . . is
going on here. In a broad sense, it made me accountable for my own education. Made me aware of the world—in my classes, as well as socially. Teachers
were real models.*

It is easy to believe as a young worker that it is necessary to pay one's dues,
to spend a certain amount of time working in the field before acquiring the
necessary skills. In many cases, the undergraduate experience provided conceptual preparation for work in human services, but only in rare cases did I
find evidence of practical training. While on-the-job training is crucial, there
are ways to equip undergraduate students with some of these skills, and many
of the people I interviewed had suggestions for very practical ways to
improve the preparation of young people for work in human services.

REDESIGNING THE CURRICULUM

When I asked these people to place themselves in the position of academics
designing curriculum, the general response was that students need hands-on
experiential learning through internships or teaching placements and the like.

I would change two central points. I would require professors to have five years of practical experience. Many of my teachers had little to no practical experience. They were theoretical without the wisdom of experience. For me, there is a difference between knowing information and experience. There must be application. Students must be regularly placed in internships where they will have hands-on experience. Without this, students will enter work without knowledge of what they are working with.

Erin, currently enrolled in a master's in social work program, elaborated on the importance of choosing internships carefully:

I think one of the most important aspects of an internship is to seriously look into the options you have—make sure that the type of work that the agency does is really what you want to be trained in. During your interview, get a clear assessment of how much and what kind of supervision you will receive. It is really beneficial if you can talk to someone who has already done an internship at that agency to get an idea of what it is like to work there. At [my university] there's a saying, "Be your own advocate"—there is truth to that saying!

It is clear that people have a strong desire for formal, structured experience and guidance, and sometimes the opportunity is not present to ask for such guidance. Erin's final exclamation sums up a key element of the experience of many young workers. For the most part, these people were trained and treated fairly well. However, it is crucial to know how to negotiate the various dynamics of working in these fields and how to be one's own advocate. So often the work of the helping professions focuses on helping the clients or consumers to gain skills and services—it is also important for workers to have access to the resources necessary to perform their own jobs comfortably. The chapters of this book explore the necessity of open communication between members of agencies and organizations.

Members of this "generation" (for lack of a better general term) have entered the workforce in an era of new theory where Total Quality Management and reengineering principles are at work. Whether or not trained formally in these principles, young people are aware of the demands on human services organizations and the relationship to private sector organizational development. It is not sufficient to simply possess certain skills and to use them to deliver services to consumers. As discussed in Chapter 2, numerous forces affect the role of each individual in an organization.

One woman offered the following comment:

I would design a program that emphasizes public policy and local government and an understanding of the role human services can and does play in an increasingly privatized economy. I'd also emphasize the importance of problem-solving skills within a dynamic and stressful field.

BALANCING ACT

I struggled daily with balancing my work and personal lives, and many of the people I interviewed expressed the same issues.

It's not just a time thing. More than that it is difficult to separate two things—problems of clients and burden of work, feeling constantly behind. We try to take time to rejuvenate at work.

As this quote from Jessica indicates, some organizations are actively aware of the potential toll and encourage workers to take time to regroup. The leadership of other organizations may not believe they have the time to spare or may be less attuned to the state of the workers, as is the case in Abby's following account.

Working for a small nonprofit taxed my body and soul. I often left work frustrated and, on some days, angry. I felt that the organization was so bogged down in the day-to-day office operations that we all ended up spinning our wheels, creating more and more paperwork. We were ineffective as an organization because of our lack of resources and because of the politics of land-use issues in a tough real estate market in a major city. Because of these hurdles, it seemed as though we, as an organization, were pushing papers around instead of enacting any real change. But, in all truthfulness, I went into the job expecting to see the effects of my work. This was unrealistic—I did not have a proper understanding of the structural forces affecting our organization and organizations like it. This affected my personal life mostly in terms of my finite amount of energy and time. There was none left for my personal life—or, I should say, not as much as I would have liked. This caused an uncomfortable merging of the two.

Clearly these issues of time and energy arise in different ways for each individual worker at any age. Each person develops his or her own method of coping with the demands of working in human services. In other cases the individual must find his or her own way to cope with the demands of this work. Daniel described his personal method.

I find meditation—or any contemplative practice like Tai Chi or yoga— incredibly important especially for caregivers because of the potential for incredible taxing on the psyche that wears all.

RESPONSIBILITY, SUPERVISION, AND SUPPORT

As described in Chapter 2, one of the most complex aspects of human services organizations is management, and the ways to manage are innumerable. Managers and supervisors in any organization struggle to find the most effective style of leadership, and this struggle can be even more complicated when it involves workers who are much younger than their supervisors. Not only are issues of level of experience and age involved, but also present is the climate in which young workers have grown up. This generation is the first to be raised in a computer-driven environment—we are almost inevitably better versed in current technology. With these habits comes the expectation of efficiency.

In their article in *Nonprofit World* (1998), Mark A. Mitchell and Robert Orwig, assistant professors of marketing and management, respectively, have laid out their own theory about workers of Generation X. While some of the generalizations made about this batch of workers seem forced, they lay out some interesting hints for working with "Xers," tips that one might argue are applicable to any group of workers, including the following:

- Make their assignments interesting and meaningful.
- Build a rich information environment, and provide plenty of feedback.
- Give them short-term projects with clear-cut goals.
- Don't just tell them what is going to happen. Tell them why.
- Spend one-on-one time with them, but be sure it's quality time. Xers hate the idea of "face time" or simply "getting your card punched."
- Avoid stereotypes and cultural insensitivity.
- Use a participatory rather than an authoritarian style.

Despite the implied kid-gloves approach to working with young people, these hints are sound and reflect the demands of the current culture. It is important for service providers to know why they are working on the projects they have been assigned. Also important is the quality of assignments and the demonstration of trust and faith in workers. One of the most common discouraging experiences recounted to me was that of young people who had entered positions where they were promised a great deal of responsibility and were subsequently left out of important organizational meetings and decisions or people who were given clerical projects when their job descriptions were "program assistants." Abby, working in an organization with only a three-person staff, expressed this frustration:

I was not given as much responsibility as I was promised. I found I had to assume the responsibility myself rather than wait for interesting projects to be given to me. I was given challenging projects, yet with all the paperwork generated by an office with no administrative assistant, I didn't have the time or energy to fully accomplish them.

I have always been conscious in my workplace of my youth and the hesitation of colleagues to trust me to complete high-level tasks, so I was interested in finding out if others had had similar experiences. Often, direct service providers felt this uneasiness in clients or in coworkers. It is difficult as a person in his or her early twenties to gain the respect of clients in these programs, especially if racial and class differences are present. I asked quite generally how these individuals felt they are or were treated as young workers in human services. Anne, who worked as a program assistant and did some work in every area of the organization that served family members of children with rare genetic diseases, responded with the following.

> *I think this question is particularly pertinent to my job. My "clients" were all parents of dying children, and they were much older than me and had much more life experience than I do. At times, I questioned if, how, and why they would turn to me for support and trust me to work with them. But they honestly never seemed to question it. So many people in the lives of these parents did not know how to be supportive. Most people have never even heard of these diseases. Many people didn't know what to say or do and subsequently did nothing. Others were so caught up in their own grief that they were not capable of giving support. So, for the most part, these parents were so glad to come into contact with anyone who was familiar with the disease, wasn't afraid to hold the children, wasn't afraid to talk about it, was capable of listening, and had the emotional energy to give to them. And I fit the requirements. They are truly the most open people I have ever met. I developed such close relationships with many of them. I don't know how they viewed me: as a daughterlike figure, a friend, a sisterlike figure, or what. But within the last month, I've had phone conversations with two of the families who both told me they loved me at the end of the conversation. And this is a year after I stopped working there. My concerns about my age had nothing to do with my ability to do the job; the concerns were only about the clients' willingness to accept me, and clearly they were able to do so despite my age.*

Also, the lack of resources and time in these not-for-profit settings can take its toll on the relationship between managers and employees. Pat, teaching in the welfare-to-work program, regrets that his supervisors did not have time or energy to train him properly.

> *The woman who was supposed to be my advisor was condescending, treated me like I knew nothing. Others trusted me that I was taking chances. Things might not work, but it was ultimately for the better. Age was a factor in class. I had to earn respect. Came in wanting to give them all the freedom, but I had to put my foot down, which was hard.*

And some of these people had very supportive mentor relationships with their supervisors.

I had the fortunate experience of working with very well-trained supervisors. They were eager to listen and explain what they had experienced and learned. I think that with openness and interest . . . I was able to feel supported and eager to learn as a young worker.

Young workers have to contend not only with age gaps between themselves and their colleagues but also in terms of clients. Clearly each situation is unique, but many factors figure in this equation. Often issues of trust and respect are in play with both employers and clients. I found that some of the older workers in my office seemed threatened by my youth. Also, all of the financial constraints and limits on staff and time resources may affect the training and treatment of young workers.

Many more questions arise after talking with these people. How do young people gain the respect of clients in service organizations? How can managers bridge the gap between themselves and young workers? These responses from workers and the principles of Chapter 2 illustrate the real need for basic communication among people in these organizations. One of the most destructive forces in a working relationship can be the sense of being silenced or not taken seriously. This potential perceived lack of agency really has little to do with the character of an entire generation. Rather, it is a natural tendency to respond more positively in an atmosphere of mutual trust and open communication. It is certainly not the sole responsibility of executive directors to keep this communication open and active.

CREATING AND COPING WITH CHANGE

The issue of change is at the core of every chapter in this book, and in these interviews I asked about two kinds of change: organizational and environmental within agencies and the social change these workers had as a goal in their human services work. As a new member of the working world trying to balance work and personal lives and all of their complications, it is easy to be swept into the culture of necessity. It is possible to believe that one can cope with change but never really be a part of effecting change or helping to initiate it. I asked individuals to comment on either type of change. No one chose to discuss change within the organization. They focused on how they were able, as individuals, to affect the lives of other individuals. Again, the responses varied.

Jessica: *It is like fighting a terrible uphill battle against systems I can't do anything about—and it's getting worse. . . . Someone got a job—one person who had every kind of problem—twenty-one years old with three kids and going to be evicted. We've come pretty far, but it's been all me and my boss fighting people. I'm controlling her life, and she would probably do it some way without me, but not in a way that is safe and effective for her and her children. It helped me learn so much and has gotten me way beyond eight months in knowledge.*

Abby: *Often I'd ask for permission and be told, "That's not how things are done." If I just went ahead and did things in a new and, what I thought, better way, it usually turned out okay that I'd changed protocol.*

While Jessica and Abby both expressed frustration about not being able to see the effects of their individual efforts, Anne was able to see daily results of her work on a small scale.

I certainly was able to make change in individuals' lives. By providing parents with resources or being the first person to truly listen to them, I was able to change their experience. Or by doing a public education event, I was able to change a family's risk of having a child with one of these diseases. But on a larger scale, I don't think I did effect change.

Pat's sense of his role in the lives of the women he taught was similar.

I really did have a sense of making change. One woman was reading every fourth word in the beginning. At the end of the program, she had read six books and was writing pretty coherently. Out of sixteen, I only had nine left at the end of the program. It made me ask, how can we keep them in here?

In contrast, Judith saw the effects of the organization's work but was not always convinced of her own contributions. Ultimately, she decided she was not the right person for the position.

I felt like the organization was making a big difference, and partly that's because they were committed to not taking any government funds. Started out in response to alcoholism, then crack epidemic hit, and they were able to change. I was on the front lines. Like the Elmer's glue you put on wood before you nail it—wouldn't hold it for long. I also feel quite strongly that the work we were doing was as much a model of learning how to be together in a functional way, and I believe that was a way of making change. I take that with me and make change. It's not measurable in a quantitative way. If a woman leaves the program without talking to anyone, I have to believe she's taking something [positive] with her.

It is clear that each individual's perception of his or her ability to effect change is dependent on many factors, including the following:

- The general effectiveness of the organization
- The individual worker's relationship to the clients
- The worker's relationship to his or her managers and colleagues

- A sense of empowerment
- Resources available to the worker and the organization
- The public attention to the particular service or issue of the work.

Each individual's sense of being able or unable to create change has a tremendous impact on his or her world view.

EMPOWERMENT AND PERSPECTIVE

Having just completed the roller coaster of the first two years after college and one year working in human services, I wanted to know how other people in similar situations were left feeling about the work they did and how their world views had been affected. Again, I was especially interested in looking at these responses in light of the current thinking about organizational management and the drive to empower workers. I asked each person to describe in general terms this "world view" and how it was affected by his or her work.

Anne, who worked with families of children with chronic illnesses, described her ambivalence.

I've really felt both ways. I definitely feel hopeful and empowered in that I've seen such incredible strength in the face of tragedy. I've seen that people can handle what they had previously considered unimaginable and that they can come out of the experience stronger; and not only stronger, but with more to offer to others. . . . However, when I think about some other issues that are more grounded in complex social causes, I get discouraged. With sexual violence, for example, there are so many things that would need to change in order to end sexual violence—sexism being the most difficult to overcome. And it's so easy to get frustrated; perhaps that's part of the reason that I've taken a break from that type of work. . . . I do intellectually believe that if we can reach one person, all of our time and energy are worth it. But when I start looking at all of the people that we couldn't reach, I get overwhelmed. Perhaps it's best to focus on small change as a goal. One way that my world view has been affected, however, is that I can truly see what's important in life. The parents that I worked with had an amazing perspective on life; they realized that the people in their lives were more important than the little things we worry about each day. I think we all know that, but they were truly able to remember that constantly. I guess it's not a privilege; they were forced to remember that constantly, but it was still a remarkable way to live.

Erin commented on this topic, too.

So far, I have found myself feeling much more passionately about the issues and populations dealt with in the field of social work. . . . I continue to feel optimistic about the work that I do and the clients I work with. I think that once you become cynical, you will not be of help to the field. The more I learn, the more I feel empowered.

Pat's comments show a general frustration with the way systems fail to serve persons in need, but she does feel a sense of personal satisfaction.

It made me aware of how much women who are underprivileged really want to get out of their situations. The view of women sitting on their asses is really ludicrous. I felt like we're in trouble. A lot of people need a lot of help and they're not getting it. People who don't have contact with this subculture really have the wrong idea. On the other hand, I felt like we, as individuals, can make an impact, effect change.

Others were more discouraged, and several persons made distinctions between personal empowerment and organizational effectiveness.

I feel more cynical because I was able to see how small one nonprofit organization can be in the face of so many larger structural powers. There needs to be a better model. Services are dependent on overworked employees and volunteers. I think the public sector needs to take up some slack. Nonprofits are providing the Band-Aids. I do feel empowered, though, because after working a year in the trenches I have a lot more perspective than I ever had and a larger understanding of the ways to effect change in the different sectors of society.

I think these quotes speak for themselves in demonstrating the complicated and exciting aspects of working in an ever-changing field. The demands of working in human services can be overwhelming. Certainly in my own working experience I have experienced both cynicism and hopefulness about the work. At any age, in any organization, challenges must be faced before work can be completed effectively.

Daniel: *Well, again, I found myself back to realizing how much good work remains to be done. I realized how listening, talking, and being with people with respect can heal people. I feel reconfirmed that these are the most helpful and beautiful acts that one person can do for another.*

Daniel's words quoted above were an unparalleled optimistic response to my question about world view, but they do echo the reasons many individuals gave for entering human services. These young people became involved in providing services because they wanted to see change happen, and they believed on some level that they would help bring about this change.

And where are these workers now in their working lives? Several people I interviewed have gone on to do completely different work, and several were inspired by their work in human services to enter social work programs, some to receive the formal and applied training that they did not receive at the undergraduate level.

Working in human services very early in their employed lives has marked each of these people.

Anne: *I had a grandparent of a child with one of these diseases tell me that for his family I was a light in an otherwise dark tunnel. That clearly meant a lot to me. Another experience that really affected me was one particular little girl who I fell in love with. Whenever possible, I would make an effort to get to the city in which she lived so that I could see her, even after I stopped working there. I was very sick for several months this past year and was unable to see her. Finally, I made arrangements to see her on February 28 of this year, but her parents canceled the trip because she was getting worse and she ended up dying on that day. I still dream about her.*

Though Mitchell and Orwig (1998) characterize Generation Xers as cynical and resentful of the burden they have been forced to adopt as a result of the irresponsible behavior of previous generations and perhaps in need of a "surrogate parent," this was not what I found during my interviews. Instead, I found a group of people whose missions were incredibly diverse, as were the results of their struggle to do good work. Each generation emerges with a new group of people eager to make change in this world, and they struggle every day with the best ways to accomplish this goal.

POINTS TO PONDER

1. While some of the subjects discussed in this chapter are unique to young people, many of the issues are the same for all workers in human services. Identify three points from this chapter that are addressed in other narrative chapters.

2. Individuals in this chapter did not always describe specific methods of coping with the difficulties or frustrations of their work. Can you imagine several concrete ways in which these issues might be addressed within the context of an organization?

CLASSROOM TO COMMUNITY

Applying the Concepts of Change

- If you have not worked in human services before, find someone who has worked in a field in which you are interested. Interview that person based on your own interests, using the general categories of this chapter as a framework: leadership, skills and training, empowerment, and world views, among others.

  If you have worked in human services, take some time to write your own narrative about your first experiences, also using the questions from this chapter as a guide.

  In both cases, consider the issues and challenges you may face in future work in human services. Think about ways in which you might address or cope with them. Consider how your current education and training will equip you for work in human services.

PREPARING FOR THE FUTURE

Chapter 14

WHERE ARE WE GOING AND HOW DO WE GET THERE?

I tend to think of the differences between leaders and managers as the differences between those who master the context and those who surrender to it.

~ Warren Bennis, Professor of Business Administration

There is little indication that the pace and complexity of change will diminish in the near future. Persons entering the field of human services, as well as those currently involved, will be confronted with a rapid succession of new technological developments, a full array of programmatic approaches—designed to address individual, family, and community needs as well as fiscal concerns—and a constantly shifting political environment in which conflicting ideologies vie for legislative and, ultimately, public support. The winds of change not only will continue to be strong but will also shift dramatically, sometimes without warning.

What can we glean from the examples in this book of how individuals and organizations involved with human services deal with change? While the descriptions of actual attempts to foster constructive change or cope with changes that have been thrust upon them may be interesting, they probably have little value for those seeking models that can be directly replicated. If these descriptions of how change has been managed are to have value, it is more likely to be at a broader, conceptual level. Taken individually and as a whole, these examples of change offer some guidance and warnings that may be useful for those engaged in human services activities. The following observations and ideas are offered with the hope that they will stimulate self-reflection and constructive action by those taking the fast-paced journey through the field of human services.

~

AND THE BEAT GOES ON

A panoramic view of the change experiences described in this book, which span nearly thirty years and a variety of human services settings, encompasses a number of consistent themes and patterns. Whether one focuses on small, relatively simple organizations, such as the Bridge Program and the nonprofit law center, or large, integrated service delivery systems, such as the state department of mental health and the Comprehensive Services Act for At Risk Youth and Families, the forces that shape change extend well beyond consideration of what will best meet the needs of consumers. External political, economic, and social factors significantly influence the nature and direction of change. Internally, personal values, leadership styles, and organizational structures and cultures often play a more critical role than demonstrated benefit or outcome in determining whether a particular program is adopted. Though different in appearance, the dynamic involved in mobilizing a broad spectrum of support to prevent a children's psychiatric hospital from being closed was essentially the same process that occurred when the secretary of health and human services brought together 145 individuals representing a wide range of constituencies to form a planning council. Ostensibly, the purpose of the planning council was to design an implementation plan for a comprehensive system of services for at risk youth and families; a less obvious but equally important purpose was to develop a statewide base to promote and support establishment of this system. In the case of the threatened closure, the goal was to protect against unwanted change; in the comprehensive services system example, the mobilization was directed at creating an innovative service system. Though the direction in relation to change was different, the strategies were similar.

It is not easy to come to grips with the fact that much of what happens in human services, including reform initiatives, is driven by nonrational forces. As the young people who had recently entered human services expressed (see Chapter 13), it was difficult to reconcile the ideal perspective of their formal educations with the actual planning and operational processes they encountered in their workplaces. By itself, awareness gained from practical experience may only lead to disillusionment. With this awareness, however, proponents of service improvement are better equipped to facilitate reform efforts.

Scanning across time and settings also provides perspective on the cyclical nature of change. For example, the political pendulum does not move continually in a fixed orbit. Rather, political ideas are colored by the particular social, cultural, economic, and technological climates in which they exist. Though similar in some respects, the political motivation for creating neighborhood-based policing in the 1970s was different from what spawned similar efforts in the 1990s. Both initiatives were intended to strengthen involvement of police officers in local communities as well as to restore citizens' confidence and trust in law-enforcement personnel. The former, however, grew out of the pervasive social unrest of the sixties while the latter has been driven much more specifically by the alarming growth of drug-related violence. In the 1970s the country was emerging from an extended period of liberal political philosophy and social activism. Police were often viewed by residents of minority and low-income communities as agents of the oppressive order who more often than not contributed negatively to the community's well-being. The primary goal of government officials during that period was to modify the public's perception of police and police departments, and those officials relied heavily on public relations strategies to accomplish this goal (Thurman, 1995). Today we are emerging from a period of political conservativism and economic prosperity. The disparity between the wealthy and the poor is greater than ever. Public officials are not only enormously embarrassed by the uncontrolled violence that exists, but they also worry about the economic and social consequences that occur when middle- and upper-class citizens flee from cities out of fear for their personal safety.

Approaches to welfare reform also have been shaped by prevailing political philosophies. In the 1960s, liberally oriented strategies to empower citizens of low-income neighborhoods, such as the community organizations efforts of Alinsky (1971), were actively supported. In the current climate of personal economic insecurity and distrust of government, reform initiatives are more concerned with removing individuals from welfare rolls than providing skills and supports to enhance self-sufficiency.

The cyclical nature of change has other implications for individuals and organizations involved in human services activities. Often people have a perception that once an obstacle has been overcome, or a problem resolved, they will no longer have to attend to the precipitating issue. Unfortunately, as the pace of change quickens the same or similar dilemma often arises within a relatively brief time interval. In the case of the children's psychiatric hospital, we saw that the changing demands of the environment made it necessary for staff to review and modify service programs on an almost continuous basis. The lull between crises also appears to be disappearing as the pace of change accelerates. In an ironic footnote, the children's psychiatric hospital, which had successfully fended off threatened closure in the 1990s, was again faced with potential calamity as this book went to press. Having adjusted to its new environment within the academic medical center, the children's psychiatric hospital was enjoying a period of programmatic success when its parent hospital modified its governance structure. This change required the larger hospital to revise the manner in which it paid for faculty services. In the process of this transformation, funding for professional staff of the children's hospital was reduced by $1 million, more than 50 percent of its total faculty budget. With the wounds of its previous trauma barely healed, hospital staff begrudgingly began mobilizing their resources to deal with this threat to the facility's survival.

BREAKTHROUGHS, TRENDS, FADS, AND OTHER FORMS OF PROGRESS

Helping individuals and organizations to deal with change has become a major industry. Consultants willing to provide technical assistance for all aspects of the change process are many. Workshops and conferences on managing change are commonplace. Entire sections in bookstores are devoted to volumes on theoretical and practical aspects of creating and coping with change (including this book).

Every burgeoning enterprise contains both sound and questionable endeavors. The change industry is no exception. The complex nature as well as the accelerated pace of the change process make it especially difficult to determine which ideas and approaches are valid and useful. In fact, one might argue that the effort to find quick fixes—a notion that is endemic to our basic beliefs about how we must deal with our fast-paced environment—is misguided because it promises something that cannot be delivered. In assessing strategies for creating and coping with change, it would be wise to look beyond the superficial appeal of trends that are currently popular and carefully examine their merits and disadvantages in relation to our intended goals. Some of the issues that deserve attention include the following.

Reinventing Reengineering

Most experts agree that successful adaptation to the current human services environment requires significant changes in the basic way in which organizations and systems operate. Since Osborne and Gaebler (1972) struck a responsive cord in their book about alternative ways in which government agencies can be more responsive and efficient in providing services, we have seen a succession of models and approaches for reforming the rigid, inefficient functioning of organizations. Few would question the need for reform; nor is there a shortage of testimony supporting some of the positive benefits that have accrued from decentralizing authority for determining how to best provide services and encouraging providers to understand and empathize with service recipients' points of view. There is, however, room for legitimate debate about whether in some instances the enormous expenditure of fiscal and human resources is justified, considering the quantitative and qualitative outcomes produced over time by many of these interventions.

The shift in popularity of organizational reform strategies illustrates the problem of continually raising the threshold for performance without adequately taking into account unintended consequences. The concept of "reinventing" organizational entities enjoyed considerable popularity during the early 1990s. By systematically assessing the effectiveness and efficiency of current practices in relation to desired outcomes, many organizations, including previously intractable bureaucratic government agencies, succeeded in making their operations more customer and outcome focused.

After a few years, administrators and organizational experts grew impatient with the pace of progress. A new generation of organizational change strategists arose, bringing with them techniques that promised quicker results. "Reinventing" was replaced by "reengineering," and many health and human services organizations stepped onto the fast track to enhance their viability within the highly competitive environment in which they were functioning. The concept made sense; the results were often disappointing. For example, an academic medical center faced with stiff competition from community hospitals that did not have associated expenses for teaching and research engaged the services of a highly respected consulting organization to assist in reducing patient-care costs. After conducting an extensive self-assessment and redesign process, the hospital adopted a plan for streamlining operations and costs. This plan had many positive features: Input from hospital staff had been extensive, the method used to identify reductions and changes had been thoughtful and systematic, and a genuine effort had been made to keep all members of the hospital community informed about the purpose and progress of the initiative. Unfortunately, the plan also had some problems.

During the consultation and planning process, the attention and energy of all upper- and middle-level management had been devoted almost exclusively to the reengineering initiative. When this phase was completed, the focus of these individuals quickly shifted to other issues. While follow-through occurred for some of the planning decisions , many of the proposed changes became lower priorities as other crises consumed the leadership of the hospital. As a result, follow-through was incomplete and monitoring of changes made did not occur as planned. In those instances where streamlining was accomplished, unintended results often came to pass. The consolidation of programs and the loss of critical personnel, many of whom took advantage of early retirement incentives, significantly reduced the knowledge and skill base of the institution and created considerable instability and disorganization. The loss of expertise and the reduction in workforce created a paradoxical effect: With fewer resources, staff became more stressed and demoralized. Their productivity diminished and, ultimately, the effectiveness and efficiency of services suffered.

The final problem with this process became apparent only after the initiative had run its course. Weighing the costs of the consultation—which were considerable—in relation to the cost savings and other benefits, some concluded that it had not been a good investment.

Harnessing Technology for the Public Good

The concept of better living through technology has been a major driving force in U.S. society since the Industrial Revolution. Occasionally we have questioned the wisdom of blind adherence to this dictum, our disillusionment with the benevolence of nuclear energy being a case in point. For the most part, however, we have maintained our faith in the ability of technology to cure ills and improve the quality of our lives.

Technology is shaping the course of human services in at least two critical ways. First, human services agencies of all sizes and shapes are traveling the fast lane on the information superhighway. Establishing automated databases, converting to electronic case records, and relying on the Internet for knowledge transfer are examples of how human services have become increasingly dependent on information technology. The advantages of this technology are obvious. The use of computers has dramatically increased the ease and speed of accessing and exchanging information. Analysis of complex data sets can be accomplished with a few strokes of a keyboard. With increased competition and advances in development, even the cost of information technology has become more reasonable.

However, as with other technological advances, potential liabilities develop. In some instances the substitution of technology has not only depersonalized service, but it also has raised concerns about confidentiality being breached due to the ease of transferring information and the absence of adequate safeguards. Information technology in some instances actually has resulted in decreased efficiency—at least for the consumer. The use of electronic telephone answering devices is a good example. Originally, these machines were intended to cut costs by utilizing machines that were less expensive to employ than human personnel. They were also intended as a means to increase access, as voice mail does. However, this technology sometimes has had the opposite effect. Anyone who has navigated through a series of computerized telephone response options to make an airline reservation or to speak to someone at a service organization ("Press 1 if you would like . . . , press 2 if you. . . .") can attest to how frustrating and inefficient these systems can be.

Innovation in information technology has virtually eliminated the time delay in communication. It is now possible to instantly transmit oral and written information to almost any point on the globe. Being able to communicate without delay has definite advantages; it also has accompanying problems or negative side effects. These unintended consequences, which we refer to as "the fax dilemma," are not as disastrous as those associated with progress in nuclear energy, but they deserve consideration as we assess how to best utilize information technology in the human services. The two most blatant side effects are (1) an increase in crisis-oriented as opposed to planned response patterns and (2) the elevated stress levels experienced by those trying to keep pace with the time demands of communication transactions. Before the fax machine, persons preparing a research or program proposal knew that the document needed to be completed several days before the deadline to allow sufficient time for transmission. While last-minute rushes to complete projects were ample, these were at least tempered by the knowledge that one could not wait until the last minute. Now with fax and Internet capability, we literally can complete a task minutes before it is due. This enhanced capacity for transmission seems to have produced a general attitude of expediency: Our time perspective for accomplishing tasks is becoming more and more compressed. As we accelerate our work pace, we often compromise thinking and review processes and, in many instances, quality and accuracy are lost. Given our tendency to acclimate to our current environment, we become desensitized to each successive increase in pace and do not pay attention to its negative effect on our physical and mental well-being.

The proliferation of communication technology has had another unintended impact on work patterns. The enormous effort required to monitor and respond to one's voice mail, e-mail, fax, pager, and cell phone, in addition to traditional written correspondence and telephone communication, serves as a major distraction for workers. A study sponsored by Pitney Bowes (1998) revealed that the average office worker sends and receives an average of 190 messages a day and is interrupted at least three times each hour by one of these communications. This constant barrage adds considerable stress to the lives of these workers; it also makes it difficult for them to concentrate on their work duties and assignments.

In addition to impacting information and communication processes, advances in technology also have a direct impact on the services people receive. Substantive advances in educational and counseling techniques, improvement in case management, and program coordination have enabled agencies to enhance the services they provide. Research in psychopharmacology and other therapeutic interventions has enhanced treatment efficacy. Recent development of critical pathway models and refinement of program evaluation methodology have added precision and accountability to the service delivery process.

While it is clear that these technological innovations have upgraded the quality of human services, the accelerated pace at which these changes are, and will be, introduced may have an unintended negative impact on human services workers and organizations.

The Polygamization of Partnership

Once upon a time, organizational life was simple. People who worked in the same organization as you were your allies. Those who worked for other agencies or corporations represented obstacles to accomplishing your task or were competitors. In today's global marketplace, the old rules have been tossed aside and replaced by new guidelines. Organizational boundaries have become fluid, and leaders in human services as well as business are encouraged to seek out relationships with other entities who may share a common interest or goal. Yesterday's competitors are today's partners, and we may be engaged in other relationships with our partners' current competitors at the same time. Unlike matrimony in Western culture, the prevailing value is that one can never have enough partnerships.

To the extent that these interorganizational relationships are productive and promote better coordination of services for individuals and families, they may be viewed as positive. Unfortunately, it is considerably easier to espouse this philosophy than to put it into practice. Successful implementation of such a complex network of relationships requires significant shifts in organizational culture and individual competence. The flexibility and sophistication required to sustain multiple, rapidly evolving interorganizational relationships cannot be attained by simply listening to a lecture or reading a book. One of the reasons that bureaucratic patterns have survived is that the predictable nature of these rote transactions has shielded workers from the vagaries of their surrounding environment. If we expect the present trend of increased linkages among organizations to produce meaningful results, we need to recognize the problems associated with actualizing this concept and make a concerted effort to address potential obstacles. The description of what happened to the Comprehensive Services Act (see Chapter 10) illustrates the difficulty of transforming philosophical principles of collaboration into actual practice. In this situation, a significant lag occurred between passage of legislation and initiation of the program and development of the interagency networks required to implement the individually tailored planning and service goals. If the movement to promote collaboration and partnership is to succeed, we need to retrain workers—both leaders and line staff—as well as redesign communication and work processes and realign incentives so that staff are rewarded rather than punished for behavior that is consistent with an organization's stated objectives. We also need to acknowledge that these tasks are not easy and will take considerable time and effort to accomplish.

Democracy Meets the Bottom Line: Seeking the Elusive Balance

Most of the current change initiatives in human services are characterized by a few common themes. In an effort to give consumers and workers greater influence in determining how services are delivered, we have introduced focus groups, quality circles, and other customer-focused processes. At the same time, the shrinking availability of resources and pressures to remain competitive have propelled organizations to institute cost-containment procedures. Occasionally these two forces converge. For instance, an organization that engages workers in finding ways to streamline service delivery without sacrificing quality is actualizing democratic principles while being sensitive to fiscal realities. More often, however, these forces diverge or, even worse, may clash with each other. This lack of fit was apparent in early managed health-care initiatives. Under enormous pressure to bring down the cost of health care, third-party payors, supported by employers, introduced procedures to limit access to care that was considered to be unnecessary. In many cases, the party determining whether a service was needed was neither a consumer nor a physician. Instead, these decisions were made by agents of insurance carriers who had direct financial interest in reducing expenditures.

After considerable public outcry from both service recipients and providers, many insurance plans have been adjusted to allow greater choice by consumers. However, while insured parties may have more choice in whom they receive services from, there are still many restrictions on the type and amount of services they are able to obtain. Some health insurance plans offer a greater range of service options if the consumer is willing to pay more for additional services.

How can we introduce change that will be responsive to both themes? Is it possible to increase consumer and worker involvement in the governance process and reduce the cost of services while also enhancing quality? The correlation between user input and quality is widely accepted; less agreement can be found about the compatibility of cost-containment and empowerment strategies and objectives. As we have seen throughout this book, complex forces cannot be successfully reconciled through simple formulaic approaches. The ecological perspective we have espoused does, however, offer some guidance about how to maintain the delicate balance among these powerful forces. The following suggestions may be useful in understanding and dealing with the multiple environmental forces that are impacting all human services organizations and programs:

• *Understand where we are in the change cycle.* In Chapter 1 we described the cyclical nature of political, social, and economic forces and how these cycles impact programmatic orientation of human services programs. Although it is not possible to predict the precise nature and duration of a particular cycle, relatively consistent patterns of evolution occur among the broad forces that shape change. For instance, within political and social domains we appear to move in either a liberal or conservative direction until the general public becomes disillusioned with or tired of that ideological position. We then move toward the opposite pole, occasionally settling at a midpoint or moderate position. The same pendular shift appears to occur in economic, organizational, and programmatic orientations. For instance, when it became apparent that environmental redesign was not a panacea, the broad-based 1960s approach to curing social ills by enhancing the environment eventually gave way to more precise interventions directed at modifying individual behavior. Likewise, reductionistic approaches to meeting human needs inevitably produce a negative reaction among consumers and the general population, thus increasing receptivity to more holistic, environmentally oriented approaches to responding to human needs. Thus we might expect the current tendency exemplified by some managed care and welfare reform initiatives to limit the amount of services provided to individuals to eventually swing toward a more holistic approach. The nature of this shift will, in large part, be determined by the prevailing political and economic situation at that time.

• *Identify and capitalize on common elements among prevailing forces.* If we can ascertain the direction in which the major forces are moving, we not only will be able to understand what is driving change, but we also may be able to harness these forces to generate changes we desire. By identifying characteristics that are shared by the prevailing political, social, and economic forces and the programmatic goals we support, we are more likely to develop effective strategies for producing positive results. For instance, knowing that current trends strongly emphasize cost containment, self-sufficiency, and program accountability, we might want to focus on competency-building and empowerment-oriented approaches that enable individuals to function effectively in work and community living settings. In our description of these programs, we would want to emphasize the long-term cost-benefit advantages of this approach.

Some risk is associated with this strategy. Being sensitive to current trends can easily become a rationalization for doing what is expedient at the expense of one's personal and professional integrity. Assessing the historical, current, and future interplay of these forces can be a useful tool as long as one does not lose sight of the basic values and goals that brought us into the field of human services.

• *Plan for the future and not the present.* With the rapid pace of change that we are experiencing, what appears to be innovative today often becomes obsolete by tomorrow. Individuals and organizations need to anticipate where political, economic, and programmatic forces are heading and develop strategies that are responsive to these directions. This often requires incremental or multiphase planning since programs and organizations rarely adapt as quickly as conceptual paradigms change.

A health-care provider organization that wants to keep pace with the demands of managed care would be shortsighted to focus solely on cost-containment measures. Having an awareness that limiting access to services is merely a stopgap measure to curtail escalating costs allows an individual or agency to look beyond the immediate crisis and prepare for future needs. The health-care organization would be wise to anticipate that successful reform requires availability of an expanded continuum of care to achieve the dual objectives of quality care and cost-efficiency. If the organization does not anticipate the need to develop alternative services and begin to work toward this goal, it is likely to fall even further behind.

• *Accept the ephemeral nature of balance.* Because political, economic, social, and programmatic forces are continually changing, finding a reasonable balance among these forces is extremely difficult. Even if one is able to achieve a position in which service quality, organizational stability, and economic considerations are reasonably accommodated, this balance is not likely to continue for any length of time due to the fluid nature of these dynamic forces. An organization may experience a reduction in funding support or a change in requirements imposed by a parent or partner organization. These demands will likely trigger a change in the internal structure of the organization that will disturb the precarious equilibrium that previously existed.

To work toward reconciling the multiple forces that impact the human services organization is admirable; to expect to achieve a lasting balance is unreasonable. Successful adaptation to change requires mental and behavioral flexibility. Not long ago, consumers and workers could expect a prolonged period of stability between changes. Today, change is the norm, and the status quo is little more than a brief episode that quickly becomes part of the individual and organizational memory bank. Unless we find a way to accept and accommodate to this evolving reality, we will most likely experience continual disappointment and frustration.

• *Is there a pony in there?* Several years ago the following joke was frequently heard at gatherings within the human services community: A young child is exhibiting unusual behavior. The parents of the child consult with a number of mental health professionals to find out what is happening with their child. Each practitioner conducts a thorough assessment but fails to come up with a plausible explanation or treatment plan. Finally, the parents contact a prominent psychologist who agrees to meet with the child at the child's home. When the psychologist arrives the child is standing in the middle of the yard next to a huge mound of manure. The psychologist observes with more than a little puzzlement as the child, who has a large shovel, frantically digs into the pile. Having exhausted all plausible hypotheses, the psychologist asks the youngster, "Why are you doing that?" Without breaking stride the child responds, "With that much horse manure, there must be a pony in there somewhere."

This joke is subject to multiple interpretations. At its most basic level, this is a story about the tenacious ability of the human mind to maintain an optimistic outlook. While some might wish to use the foul-smelling mound in the story as a metaphor for the changes we are experiencing in human services, it might be more appropriate to ask whether this frenetic change activity we are engaged in will produce a result that is nearly as favorable as that which the child believed would be found inside the pile of manure.

SHAPING ONE'S PERSPECTIVE

To the extent that reality is in the eye of the beholder, each individual's view of the future is influenced by long-standing personal attributes as well as recent experience and those few tangible indicators that are used to forecast the future. Given the enormity of the forces that shape policy and practice and the general sense of helplessness that accompanies the whirlwind pace of change we are experiencing, it is not surprising that many of us feel a need to put these events into perspective. Often we are inclined to turn to familiar and comfortable sources to help us make sense of what is currently happening and where these changes in human services will take us. Some people rely primarily on spiritual guidance; others favor more empirical approaches. Many individuals utilize a combination of these approaches. Whichever framework one employs, successful adaptation requires the formulation of a clear, comprehensive perspective on how to best approach the daunting change process that individuals and institutions in human services currently experience. Although the content of each person's framework will be uniquely suited to his or her interests, beliefs, and knowledge, that perspective needs to incorporate certain critical elements. Included among the questions that need to be addressed in developing one's perspective on change and human services are the following:

1. *Is the current course of change likely to enhance or impede our ability to promote growth and self-sufficiency, prevent problems, strengthen communities and families, and assist those who are experiencing deprivation and disability?* There is no shortage of opinion on whether our current course is desirable or despicable. Persons who share the traditionally liberal orientation toward human services—clearly the majority of human services workers and consumers—are noticeably anxious about the trends of reducing government involvement and fiscal support. Those who have faith in technology and wish to see greater accountability tend to think that we are moving in the right direction. Until crystal-ball technology is perfected, the probability of accurately predicting where human services will be in ten or twenty years is low. In the absence of a valid forecasting instrument, each of us constructs a future scenario based on long-standing personal beliefs as well as subjective interpretation of the anticipated interplay among the major forces that shape change. In some ways the specific content of our view of the future is less important than the existence of a coherent perspective.

2. *Which strategies are most likely to yield changes in the desired direction?* This question can be asked at several levels. At the macro level we can speculate on grand political, social, and economic strategies that might shift the balance of our society's priorities toward compassion and caring rather than personal acquisition and competition. More relevant is how each of us approaches our own circumscribed situation: our relationship to those we serve, the organization in which we function, the community in which we live. Given that the particular shape and size of one's personal domain will dictate which strategies are most appropriate, several principles may be useful in formulating personal strategies for influencing change. These include the following:

a. Effective change in complex situations requires a multistrategy approach.

b. On the other hand, trying to change too many things at once is likely to make things worse. The advice given to runners preparing for a long-distance race seems applicable. Coaches often tell individuals getting ready for a long race to focus on increasing speed or distance but not both simultaneously. The dual-pronged training approach has the appeal of being more efficient but often leads to injuries that prevent the runner from even getting to the starting line. By establishing priorities, beginning with aspects of change that may be easier to accomplish, one is able to proceed in a rational and orderly fashion while also building confidence and momentum needed for more daunting challenges.

3. *What is a reasonable time frame for achieving change?*   Change takes time; meaningful change takes a long time. One common mistake made by persons engaged in change is to assume that once the organizational structure is altered, the desired substantive changes, including staff performance and pro-grammatic direction, will occur automatically. Change typically proceeds in sequential fashion. Changing the organizational structure can be accom-plished relatively quickly. Altering mechanical tasks or duties may take longer but can be accomplished in a relatively short period. Programmatic modifi-cations are usually more complex and require a longer period of gestation. The most difficult area of change is the culture of the organization. Modify-ing work ethics and communication patterns requires patience and tenacity. Long after last year's reorganization or redesign initiative has been replaced by a newer version, workers tenaciously cling to their territorial habits.

4. *What can I do to survive all these changes?*   With the trend toward down-sizing and the accelerating pace at which change is occurring, participants in the human services system are experiencing greater levels of stress. Although nearly everyone has adapted by working harder, sheer effort alone does not ensure that workers will be productive and effective. Becoming familiar with technology and learning efficient work habits is necessary, but finding ways to take care of one's self is just as important. Having a reasonable perspective on what one can influence is helpful. Finding ways to buffer and reduce stress increases longevity and satisfaction. Making a clear distinction between work and the rest of life is also important.

Addressing these questions may be useful for someone who is grappling with the complexities of the current human services environment and the direction in which it is moving. Successful completion of this exercise will not, however, automatically yield a balanced perspective on change. Trying to make sense of what is happening and how one can exert a constructive influence is an ongoing process characterized by periods of relative clarity as well as confusion. A good perspective generally is one that keeps us moving in a consistent direction but allows us the flexibility to adjust our course of action to respond to changing conditions.

5. *Where's the government?* It is not possible to have a serious discussion about human services without addressing the role of government. In spite of the current trend toward government bashing, ensuring that individuals, especially those who are physically, economically, and socially vulnerable, receive services that are responsive to their needs will require that government play a significant role. As Marian Wright Edelman points out in her eloquent treatise *The Measure of Our Success: A Letter to My Children and Yours* (1993), "It is a dangerously short-sighted nation that fantasizes absolute self-sufficiency as the only correct way of life. Throughout our history, we have given government help to our people and then have forgotten that fact when it came time to celebrate our peoples' achievements."

The question we should be addressing is not whether government should be involved but what role it should play and how this role should be performed. Current trends lean strongly toward privatization. The private sector has the competence and flexibility to deliver services more efficiently than government agencies. The real issue is whether the private sector is interested in and capable of responding to our most pressing challenges. For example, it is relatively easy to establish a preventive health-care system for families with good health status and reliable sources of income and health insurance. Health-maintenance organizations (HMOs) and other types of health-care providers have demonstrated that they can provide decent preventative and maintenance care as well as occasional acute care and still make a profit. There is more room for debate on the issue of whether the needs of persons with multiple chronic problems can be adequately served by the private sector. The intensity and duration of effort required and the difficulty of finding funding sources that offer an adequate financial margin make this latter population much less appealing.

Even if the government finds sufficient financial incentives to convince private agencies to serve persons with the greatest needs, only the government can play certain other critical roles. In spite of the present antagonism toward increasing taxes, government will most likely continue to be the primary funding source for services provided to those who have no other way to pay for them. The debate about who should be responsible for paying for these services—local, state, or federal government—shall probably continue indefinitely and the locus of responsibility may shift, but ultimately the fiscal burden will continue to reside with one government agency or another.

Government will also continue to be responsible for some aspects of monitoring and regulation. Government credibility and popularity are currently low in regard to these functions. And there is considerable opportunity for developing alternative mechanisms for assessing whether services are adequate, such as peer and consumer review using outcome-based performance measures. In time, public sentiment will probably change. Whether the public tires of the current political rhetoric or becomes less tolerant of our insensitivity to those who are most in need, the public will eventually demand greater accountability for the programmatic and financial aspects of human services. Who else but the government is able to perform the critical functions of protecting the rights of vulnerable consumers and ensuring that the money of taxpayers is used for the purposes it was intended?

It is unrealistic as well as unwise to advocate for a return to traditional government functioning. To argue that government has a legitimate role to play in promoting, supporting, and regulating human services is reasonable and timely.

ALL POLITICS AND ALMOST ALL CHANGE ARE PERSONAL

Throughout this book we have stressed the importance of developing a constructive perspective on change. We have emphasized the need to understand the political, economic, social, cultural, and technological forces that shape change and to not overpersonalize our reaction to the changes that occur in our immediate environment. A comprehensive and rational perspective and an ability to take care of one's self are essential survival skills in the current fast-paced human services environment.

Having reiterated these messages ad nauseam, we wish to end this book with a seemingly paradoxical message. No matter how much one tries to depersonalize the dynamics of change, it is difficult to avoid the conclusion that change is inevitably experienced at a personal level and that the course of change is heavily influenced by personal factors. Organizational decisions are clearly impacted by the personalities of organizational leaders. Efforts to restructure and downsize agencies and corporations have had an enormous impact on the personal lives of workers and their families. For individuals who have been laid off or downgraded, the economic, social, and psychological consequences have been obvious and painful. Even those whose jobs have not been directly affected often experience negative side effects such as the phenomenon of survivor's guilt that occurs among persons who retain their jobs after reductions in the workforce. Also, recipients of service have a considerable personal stake in the change process. Virtually all modifications in the organization, funding, and provision of services have a direct personal impact on consumers.

Providing individuals who experience change with a clear understanding of the rationale and purpose of change is necessary but not sufficient. People want to know how change will affect them personally. An organization restructuring its service delivery system is less likely to experience resistance from employees who have a clear sense of their new roles and their place within the new structure than is an organization that has not sufficiently responded to personal concerns of staff. When service recipients are told directly how changes will personally impact them, they are better able to adapt, even when the new arrangements are viewed as less favorable than the status quo.

How can we reconcile these seemingly contradictory messages about the personalization of change? Convincing arguments can be made supporting the importance of establishing a rational perspective to aid planning, implementation, and adaptation to change. At the same time it is difficult to deny that personal factors invariably play a part in the change process. Like most other issues related to change in human services, developing a reasonable perspective on how to anticipate, understand, and appropriately respond to personal dynamics is a complex endeavor. Whether one is dealing with an individual, organization, service system, or community, the following guidelines may be useful in dealing with the personal elements of change:

• Be aware of your own or others' possible reactions to all phases of change. This includes proactive initiatives to create change as well as efforts to adapt to the consequences of change efforts.

• Incorporate into the planning process an awareness that individuals are primarily concerned with how change will affect them personally. This issue should be addressed as early and directly as possible. It is useful to inform employees about why a particular change is being enacted. However, unless we provide information about their concrete concerns to the staff involved, such as how their day-to-day work activities will be impacted and who their supervisor will be, these individuals will remain preoccupied with these concerns and will probably not pay attention to more global discussions of the purpose and benefits of change.

• Even though all organizations should be sensitive to the needs of its employees, be even more aware of and responsive to the feelings, concerns, and well-being of the workforce in the human services community. Although economic and political forces exert a strong influence on the provision of human services, be careful not to underestimate the role of personal factors. An unhappy workforce is unlikely to be responsive to the needs of its clientele. Conversely, staff who feel respected and supported are more likely to genuinely care for and empower consumers even when resources are not plentiful. Consistent with the axiom that a little knowledge is dangerous, do not allow your understanding of the impact of external forces on human services to lull you into a passive posture regarding your ability to influence the nature of quality and services. You may not be able to directly modify the external forces impinging on human services, but you can utilize the knowledge and skills you employ with clients to enhance the human services workplace. If you respond constructively to the concerns and needs of staff, you are likely to have a positive impact on their attitudes and motivational state. Enhanced worker satisfaction is likely to translate into a more energetic, cohesive workforce. A human services system staffed by such a team is much more likely to succeed in responding to and empowering the individuals and families that they serve.

In developing a balanced perspective on change within the human services, always consider the personal element. Understanding and taking into account the impact of change on individuals, as well as developing strategies for assisting persons to accept and adapt to change, are critical to the success of any change initiative. Beyond the immediate utilitarian value of addressing the impact of change on human services consumers and workers, at least one other compelling reason merits paying attention to the personal element. Much of the impetus for change initiatives has been aimed at improving performance in such areas as efficiency, productivity, and customer satisfaction. The initiatives cited in this book and others have demonstrated that these are achievable objectives. The question that must be addressed in the future is how much can we expect from change?

As expectations are continually raised and the pace of everyday life accelerates, we will eventually reach a point of diminishing returns. Although considerable potential to expand our technological capacity remains, the capacity of human beings to cope effectively with increased stress is certainly more limited. How much faster can people work? How many changes can they endure before "burning out"? At what point does organizational instability produced by constant change become detrimental to accomplishing the objectives for which these changes were designed?

Just as it became necessary to impose speed limits when technological advances made it possible for motor vehicles to move more quickly, shouldn't we also be studying the dangers associated with organizational change and considering ways to monitor and control the course of change? We need to acknowledge that the potential for improving performance and enhancing services is directly dependent on our ability to harness this powerful vehicle. If we persist in accelerating the pace of change, we run the risk of wearing out staff. Without an energetic, motivated workforce, the human services system is unlikely to be responsive to the needs of those for whom the services are intended. If we hope to actualize our vision of a comprehensive and compassionate human services delivery system, we need to temper the current fast-paced, economically and technologically driven course of change with a more person-oriented approach. Genuine reform requires us to embrace a philosophy and an accompanying set of strategies that recognize the value and vulnerability of our human resources and keep us focused on the real reason we chose to become involved in the field of human services.

POINTS TO PONDER

1. Which of the emerging forces and trends that exist in today's society are most likely to influence the future course of human services and what will be their probable impact? Consider specific developments within human services as well as broader political, economic, social, cultural, and technological trends.

2. The importance of developing a balanced perspective has been emphasized throughout this book. Understanding the individual forces that shape change as well as how these forces interact with each other is a prerequisite for making sense of the changes that are taking place and developing strategies to produce desirable outcomes. What knowledge and skills do individuals need to successfully develop a reasonable and comprehensive perspective on the dynamics of change in human services at the individual, organizational, and systems levels?

3. The complex nature and frenetic pace of today's human services system can take a serious toll on participants—both consumers and staff. To function well and survive in this hectic environment, individuals must learn how to cope with the stress and confusion that accompany change. What are some useful strategies individuals can employ to deal with stress and frustration in this rapidly changing environment? What specific cognitive or behavioral approaches might enable individuals to prevent or reduce stress while also enabling them to function more effectively?

4. Describe the human services system of the year 2025. How will it be different from today's services system and what will account for those changes? Who will provide services, how will they be provided, and how will they be paid for?

CLASSROOM TO COMMUNITY

Applying the Concepts of Change

- Identify a human services organization or system whose programs are being threatened by changes in the human services environment. Design a strategy for strengthening this group's effectiveness and viability. Establish goals and outcomes the organization might strive for, and develop an action plan for achieving these goals in the next one to five years. Discuss the various forces that may influence the organization's course of development, and describe how you would deal with each of these in your planning initiative.

- Interview a recipient or provider of human services. Ask this individual to describe the stresses experienced in the human services environment and how he or she copes with them.

REFERENCES

Adams, P., and Krauth, K. (1995). "Working with Families and Communities: The Patch Approach," in P. Adams and K. Nelson, *Reinventing Human Services: Community- and Family-centered Practice.* Hawthorne, NY: Aldine deGruyter.

Adams, P., and Nelson, K., eds. (1995). *Reinventing Human Services: Community- and Family-centered Practice.* Hawthorne, NY: Aldine deGruyter.

Alinsky, S. (1971). *Rules for Radicals.* New York: Vintage Books.

Apter, S.J. (1982). *Troubled Children/Troubled Systems.* Elmsford, NY: Pergamon Press.

Apter, S.J., Apter, D.S., Trief, P.M., Cohen, N., Woodlock, D., and Harootunian, B. (1978). *The Bridge Program: Comprehensive Psychoeducational Services for Troubled Children and Families.* Syracuse, NY: Syracuse University School of Education.

Bennis, W. (1989). *On Becoming a Leader.* Reading, MA: Addison-Wesley Publishing.

Bickman, L., and Rog, D.J., eds. (1998). *Handbook of Applied Social Research Methods.* Thousand Oaks, CA: Sage Publications.

Blake, R.B., and Mouton, J.S. (1994). *The Managerial Grid,* 4th ed.. Houston: Gulf Publishing.

Bowditch, J.L., and Buono, A. (1985). *A Primer on Organizational Behavior.* New York: John Wiley and Sons.

Bratton, W., with Knobler, P. (1998). *Turnaround: How America's Top Cop Revised the Crime Epidemic.* New York: Random House.

Campbell, J. (1990). *The Hero's Journey: The World of Joseph Campbell.* San Francisco: Harper & Row.

Carling, D.J. (1995). *Return to Community: Building Support Systems for People with Psychiatric Disabilities.* New York: Guilford Press.

Champy, J. (1995). *Reengineering Management: A Mandate for New Leadership.* New York: Harper Business.

Cohen, R., Singh, N.N., Hosick, J., and Tremaine, L. (1992). "Implementing a Responsive System of Mental Health Services for Children," *Clinical Psychology Review,* 12, 819–28.

Covey, S.R. (1990). *The Seven Habits of Highly Effective People: Restoring the Character Ethic.* New York: Simon & Schuster.

Deming, W.E. (1982). *Quality, Productivity and Competitive Position.* Cambridge, MA: Massachusetts Institute of Technology, Center for Advanced Engineering Study.

_____ (1986). *Out of Crisis.* Cambridge, MA: Massachusetts Institute of Technology, Center for Advanced Engineering Study.

Drucker, P.F. (1990). *Managing the Non-profit Organization: Practices and Principles.* New York: HarperCollins.

_____ (1992). *Managing for the Future: The Nineties and Beyond.* New York: Dutton.

_____ (1993). *Concept of the Corporation.* New Brunswick, NJ: Transaction Publishers.

_____ (1995). *Managing in a Time of Great Change.* New York: Truman Talley Books/Dutton.

Edelman, M.W. (1993). *The Measure of Our Success: A Letter to My Children and Yours.* New York: HarperCollins.

Fayol, H., trans. from the French edition by C. Storrs. (1949). *General and Industrial Management.* London: Pitman.

Fosler, R.S. (1990). *Demographic Change and the American Future.* Pittsburgh, PA: University of Pittsburgh Press.

Gantt, H.L. (1974). *Organizing for Work.* Easton, PA: Hive Publishing Co.

Hammer, M., and Champy, J. (1993). *Reengineering the Corporation: A Manifesto for Business Revolution.* New York: Harper Business.

Hargrove, E.C., and Glidewell, J.C. (1990). *Impossible Jobs in Public Management.* Lawrence: University of Kansas Press.

Hersey, P., and Blanchard, K.H. (1969). "Life Cycle Theory of Leadership," *Training and Development Journal,* 23:5, 26–34.

Hersey, P., Blanchard, K.H., and Johnson, P. (1996). *Management of Organizational Behavior: Utilizing Human Resources,* 7th ed. Upper Saddle River, NJ: Prentice-Hall.

Himmelstein, D.U., Woolhandler, S., and Wolfe, S.M. (1992). "The Vanishing Health Care Safety Net: New Data on Uninsured Americans," in *International Journal of Health Services,* 22, 381–96.

Huse, E.F. (1980). *Organizational Development and Change.* St. Paul, MN: West Publishing Company.

Ishikawa, K., trans. by D.J. Lu. (1985). *What Is Total Quality Control? The Japanese Way.* Englewood Cliffs, NJ: Prentice-Hall.

Joe, T. (1984). "Shredding an Already Tattered Safety Net, in Weicher, T., ed. *Maintaining the Safety Net: Redistribution Programs in the Reagan Administration.* Washington, DC: American Enterprise Institute for Public Policy Research.

Joint Commission on the Mental Health of Children (1969). *Crisis of Child Mental Health.* New York: Harper and Row.

Kane, R.L., ed. (1997). *Understanding Health Care Outcomes Research.* Gaithersburg, MD: Aspen Publishers.

Kao, H.S.R., Sinha, D., and Sek-Hong, N., eds. (1995). *Effective Organizations and Social Value.* New Delhi, India: Sage Publications India, PVT LTD.

Katzenbach, J.R., and the RCL Team (1995). *Real Change Leaders: How You Can Create Growth and High Performance at Your Company.* New York: Random House.

Kretzmann, J.P., and McKnight, J.L. (1993). *Building Communities from the Inside Out: A Path Toward Funding and Mobilizing a Community's Assets.* Chicago: ACTA Publications.

Kubler-Ross, E. (1981). *Living with Death and Dying.* New York: Macmillan.

Kunnes, R. (1994). "Vision: Behavioral Healthcare Mega-Trends (or the End of Managed Care as We Know It)," in *Behavioral Healthcare Tomorrow.*

Lader, M.H., and Herrington, R. (1996). *Biological Treatments in Psychiatry.* Oxford, England: Oxford University Press.

Lamb, H.R., and Associates (1976). *Community Survival for Long-term Patients.* San Francisco: Jossey-Bass Publishers.

Levine, M., and Levine, A. (1970). *A Social History of Helping Services; Clinics;,Courts, School, and Community.* New York: Appleton-Century-Crofts.

Levine, M., and Perkins, D.V. (1997). *Principles of Community Psychology: Perspectives and Applications,* 2nd ed. New York: Oxford University Press.

Lyons, J., Howard, R.I., O'Mahoney, M.T., and Lish, J.O. (1997). *The Measurement and Management of Clinical Outcomes in Mental Health.* New York: John Wiley and Sons.

MacBeth, G. (1993). "Collaboration Can Be Elusive: Virginia's Experience in Developing an Interagency System of Care" in Administration and Policy in Mental Health, 20:4, 259–81.

Means, R., and Smith, R. (1994). *Community Care: Policy and Practice.* Houndmills, Basingstoke, Hampshire: Macmillan.

Metcalf, H.C., and Hurwick, L. (1942). *Dynamic Administration: The Collected Works of Mary Parker Follett.*

Mitchell, M.A., and Orwig, R. (1998). "Generation X: How to Manage, Market, and Motivate Them," in *Nonprofit World*, 16, 1, 36–41.

Moss, M.A. (1996). *Applying TQM to Product Design and Development*. New York: M. Decker.

O'Donohue, and Krasner, L., eds. (1995). *Theories of Behavior Therapy: Exploring Behavior of Change*. Washington, DC: American Psychological Association.

Olfson, M. (1990). "Assertive Community Treatment: An Evaluation of the Experimental Evidence," in *Hospital and Community Psychiatry*, 41, 634–41.

Oliver, T.R. (1998). "The Collision of Economics and Politics in Medicaid Managed Care: Reflections on the Course of Change in Maryland," in *Milbank Quarterly*, 176, 1, 59–101.

Omachonou, V.K, and Ross, J.E. (1994). *Principles of Total Quality*. Stillray Beach, FL: St. Lucy Press.

Osborne, D., and Gaebler, T. (1972). *Reinventing Government: How the Entrepreneurial Spirit Is Transforming the Public Sector*. Reading, MA: Addison-Wesley Publishing.

Osborne, D., and Plastrik, P. (1997). *Banishing Bureaucracy: The Five Strategies for Reinventing Government*. Reading, MA: Addison-Wesley Publishing.

Parmelee, D.X., ed. (1996). *Child and Adolescent Psychiatry*. St. Louis, MO: Mosby.

Peters, T.J. (1994). *The Pursuit of Wow!: Every Person's Guide to Topsy-turvy Times*. New York: Vintage Books.

Peters, T.J., and Austin, N. (1985). *A Passion for Excellence: The Leadership Difference*. New York: Random House.

Peters, T.J., and Waterman, R.H. (1982). *In Search of Excellence: Lessons from America's Best-run Companies*. New York: Harper and Row.

Pitney Bowes' Work Place Communications in the 21st Century (1998). Stamford, CT: Pitney Bowes Incorporated.

The President's Commission on Mental Health (1978). *Task Panel Reports Submitted to the President's Commission on Mental Health*. Washington, DC: U.S. Government Printing Office.

Rutter, M. (1990). "Psychosocial Resilience and Protective Mechanisms," in M.J. Rolf, A.S. Masten, and D. Cicchetti, eds., *Risk and Protective Factors in the Development of Psychopathology*. New York: Cambridge University Press.

Schorr, L.B. (1994). "Children: The Endangered Species," paper presented at the forum entitled Children: The Endangered Species, Boone, NC: Appalachian State University.

Schorr, L.B. (1997). *Common Purpose: Strengthening Families and Neighborhoods to Rebuild America*. New York: Doubleday.

Schorr, L.B., and Schorr, D. (1988). *Within Our Reach: Breaking the Cycle of Disadvantage*. New York: Anchor Books, Doubleday.

Shellenbarger, S. (1993). "Work Study Finds Loyalty Is Weak, Divisions of Race and Gender Are Deeper," in *Wall Street Journal*, September 10, 1993.

Sherman, V.C. (1993). *Creating the New American Hospital.* San Francisco: Jossey-Bass Publishers.

Singh, N.N., ed. (1997). *Prevention and Treatment of Severe Behavior Problems: Models and Methods in Developmental Disabilities.* Pacific Grove, CA: Brooks/Cole.

Smale, G.G., with Tuson, G. (1992). *Managing Change Through Innovation: Towards a Model for Developing and Reforming Social Work Practice and Social Service Delivery.* London: National Institute for Social Work.

Stein, L.I., and Test, M.S. (1980). "Alternative to Mental Hospital Treatment: I. Conceptual Model, Treatment Program, and Clinical Evaluation," in *Archives of General Psychiatry,* 37, 392–97.

Stoesz, D., and Karger, H.J. (1996). "Suffer the Children," in *The Washington Monthly,* 28, 6, 20–25.

Stone, D. (1997). *Policy Paradox: The Art of Political Decision Making.* New York: W.W. Norton and Company.

Stroul, B.A., ed. (1996). *Children's Mental Health: Creating Systems of Care in a Changing Society.* Baltimore: P.H. Brookes Publishing.

Taylor, F.W. (1911). *The Principles of Scientific Management.* New York: Harper and Brothers.

Thurman, H.C. (1995). "Community Policing: The Police as a Community Resource," in P. Adams and K. Nelson, *Reinventing Human Services: Community and Family-centered Practice.* Hawthorne, NY: Aldine deGruyter.

Tomlinson, D., and Carrier, J., eds. (1996). *Asylum in the Community.* London: Routledge.

Torrey, E.F. (1997). *Out of the Shadows: Confronting America's Mental Illness Crisis.* New York: John Wiley and Sons.

Tucker, R.B. (1991). *Managing the Future: The Essential Survival Tools for Business in Today's Market.* New York: Berkeley Books.

U.S. Bureau of Labor Statistics (1998). *Number of Jobs, Labor Market Experience and Earnings Growth: Results from a Longitudinal Survey.* Washington, DC: U.S. Department of Labor. Internet: http://www.bls.gov/news.release/nlsoy.toc.htm.

U.S. Bureau of the Census (1993). *Statistical Abstract of the United States, 1993,* 113th ed. Washington, DC: U.S. Department of Commerce.

United States Office of Technology Assessment (1986). "Children's Mental Health: Problems and Services—A Background Paper." Washington, DC: U.S. Government Printing Office.

Virginia Department of Planning and Budget (1990). *Study of Children's Residential Care Services.* Richmond, VA: Virginia Department of Planning and Budget.

Weiss, C. H. (1972). *Evaluating Action Programs: Readings in Social Action and Education.* Boston: Allyn and Bacon.

Yoe, J.T., Santarcangelo, S., Atkins, M., and Buchard, J.D. (1996). "Wrap-around Care in Vermont: Program Development, Implementation and Evaluation of a Statewide System of Individualized Services," in *Journal of Child and Family Studies,* 5, 23–37.

INDEX